the New AbsDiet Cookbook

Hundreds of Powerfood Meals That Will Flatten Your Stomach and Keep You Lean for Life!

DAVID ZINCZENKO

EDITORIAL DIRECTOR of Men'sHealth & Women'sHealth *With Jeff Csatari*

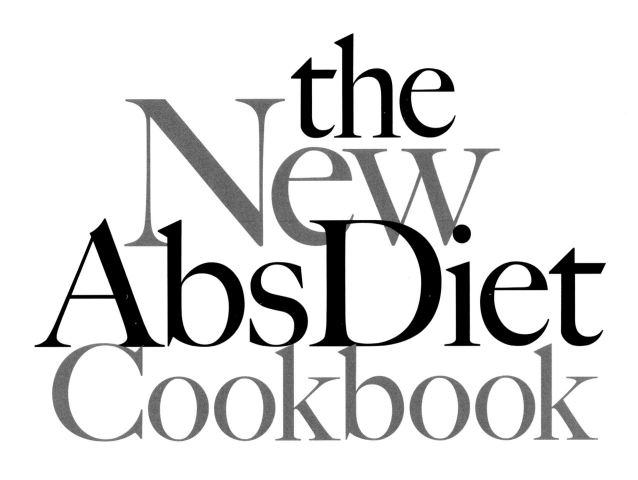

the New Abs Diet Cookbook

© 2010 by Rodale Inc.

Rodale books may be purchased for business or promotional use or for special sales. For information, please write to:
Special Markets Department, Rodale, Inc., 733 Third Avenue, New York, NY 10017

Men's Health and *Women's Health* are registered trademarks of Rodale Inc.

Printed in the United States of America

Rodale Inc. makes every effort to use acid-free ⊗, recycled paper ♻.

Photographs by Mitch Mandel/Rodale Images
Photo editing by Tara Long
Book design by John Lin with George Karabotsos, design director, *Men's Health* Books
Cover design inspired by Joe Heroun
Food stylist: Melissa Reiss, except for
images on pages 106, 163, 187, 190, 193, 194, 216, 219, 224, 228, 232, 236, 240 by Diane Simone Vezza
Process illustrations by Bradley R. Hughes
Icon illustrations by L-Dopa

Library of Congress Cataloging-in-Publication Data

The abs diet cookbook : hundreds of power-food meals that will flatten your stomach and keep you lean for life / David Zinczenko, editor-in-chief of Men's Health, with Jeff Csatari.

p.   cm.

Includes index.
ISBN-13: 978-1-60529-277-9 (direct)
ISBN-10: 1-60529-277-X (direct)
ISBN-13: 978-1-60529-314-1 (trade)
ISBN-10: 1-60529-314-8 (trade)

1. Reducing diets.   2. Reducing diets—Recipes.   3. Nutrition.
4. Abdominal exercises.   I. Csatari, Jeff.   II. Title.

RM222.2.Z558 2010

641.5'635—dc22   2009053335

2 4 6 8 10 9 7 5 3 1   hardcover

We inspire and enable people to improve their lives and the world around them

For more of our products visit **rodalestore.com** or call 800-848-4735

www.absdietonline.com

To men and women everywhere who are ready to take up arms—
or at least a spatula—to battle America's obesity crisis. We'll win this war,
one belly at a time.

Contents

Acknowledgments

There were lots of cooks in the kitchen during the preparation of this book. But for once that's a good thing, and I'd like to extend my heartfelt thanks to all those who rolled up their sleeves. In particular:

Maria Rodale and the rest of the Rodale family, whose support, encouragement, and inspiration are behind every product Rodale Inc. brings to you.

The entire *Men's Health* and *Women's Health* editorial staffs—the smartest, most innovative, and hardest-working group of writers, editors, researchers, designers, photo directors, and Web masters in the industry.

Steve Perrine, editor-in-chief of Men's Health Books; George Karabotsos, design director, and Joe Heroun, whose collective design handiwork can be seen on the cover; John Lin, who designed the inside pages; Debbie McHugh, who made sure we made our deadlines; Sophie Fitzgerald for providing nutrition analysis; and my coauthor, Jeff Csatari.

A huge thank you to the Rodale books team: Karen Rinaldi, Chris Krogermeier, Sara Cox, Erin Williams, Brooke Meyers, Jean Rogers, and Lisa Ternullo; to illustrators L-Dopa and Bradley R. Hughes; and to food wizards Tara Long, Melissa Reiss, and Diane Simone Vezza, and photographer Mitch Mandel for their amazing talent for bringing the recipes to life through the photography in this book.

Special thanks to my brother, Eric, whose relentless teasing drove me to make fitness a priority in my life.

And to my mother, Janice, whose love and support have made everything possible.

And last but not least, to everyone who contributed to this book by sampling our recipes, over and over and over again. The Tums are on me.

Introduction

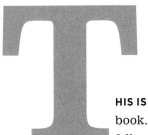

HIS IS NOT YOUR standard cookbook. A simple flip through the following pages will tell you that. Among the words you will not find in these pages: au jus, glacée, ragout, béchamel, bouquet garni, and coq au vin.

Among the words you will find in the following pages: lean, abs, strong, fit, healthy, body.

What you're holding in your hands is not just a compilation of food tips and smart recipes: *The New Abs Diet Cookbook* is, in fact, a training manual—one that will help you to strip away fat (from your belly first!); build lean, strong muscle; boost your energy level; and discover the flat, firm abdomen hiding beneath the softer layers of your midsection.

Of course, traditional cookbooks have their place on the kitchen shelf. Sometimes you need to find a pumpkin pie recipe, learn the best way to braise a capon, or figure out what to do with the catch of the day. But most cookbooks are training tools for your tastebuds. *The New Abs Diet Cookbook* is a training tool for your whole body, one that will reshape your physique into a tower of lean, sexy muscle. (And your tastebuds are going to get pretty buff, too!)

Now, you might be thinking: How can eating delicious food help me to become leaner and fitter? How can a cookbook help me build muscle and get rid of my gut? After all, isn't building muscle just a matter of going to the gym and throwing around heavy objects? And isn't shedding flab just a matter of eating less and trading in cupcakes for rice cakes?

Well, no. Shedding belly fat isn't just about eating less food, and building muscle isn't just about going to the gym and dripping sweat on all the gleaming chrome machinery. The groundwork for both goals is laid right in your own kitchen. And that's where this book comes in. By centering all of the recipes around the 12 Abs Diet Powerfoods—the most powerful fat-burning, muscle-building, disease-fighting foods known to man—this cookbook will do more than simply keep you happy and well-fed. It will help you strip away fat (did I mention from your belly first?), up to 20 pounds in the next 4 to 6 weeks. And you will never, ever go hungry—or eat a single rice cake.

How to Rediscover Your Abs

When you think about uncovering your abs, it's easy to get discouraged. The only people we ever see with abs seem to be celebrities and models, and it's a lot easier to keep your belly flat when movie studios are investing millions of dollars in your midsection. So it's not hard to fall into the mistaken belief that unless you have a personal trainer, a 2,000-square-foot home gym, a nutritionist on call, and an entourage of masseuses, abs are just plain out of reach. You look down at your spare tire—and look up at the mountain of work and family obligations coming at you each day—and think, "My abs are gone, and I'll never see them again."

But I'm here to tell you that you're wrong.

How do I know? Because helping you find your abs is my job.

As editor-in-chief of *Men's Health*, editorial director of *Women's Health*, and author of the bestselling *Eat This, Not That!* book series, I've been analyzing health, fitness, and nutrition information for the better part of two decades. In that time, I've seen diet and exercise fads come and go. (Remember the low-fat craze? The low-carb craze? The cabbage soup diet?) I've tried every kind of exercise equipment, talked to all of the leading researchers in the nutrition and fitness fields, and crunched the numbers on studies (and a number of studies on crunches!) to find the most effective ways to build the lean, flat abs that my readers are searching for.

And what I've learned from all that research—beyond the fact that cabbage soup tastes really, really bad—is that finding your abs is possible. And it's not as hard as you'd think, even if you've struggled with weight issues all your life.

Indeed, when I wrote *The Abs Diet* back in 2004, I knew that all the research we had done at *Men's Health* would yield the easiest, most effective weight-loss plan imaginable. And I was right. *The Abs Diet* and *The Abs Diet for Women* have sold more than 3 million copies and been translated into 30 languages. (We recently updated both books—*The New Abs Diet* and *The New Abs Diet for Women*—with the latest nutrition and fitness research, useful tips, advice, and workouts for even faster results.) What these millions of Abs Diet readers have discovered is the same thing that you'll discover: Your abs aren't extinct. They're just waiting for you to find them again.

Where Abs Await

Think of your abdominal muscles as long-lost pals you once knew in high school. Sure, when you were younger, you used to see them every day, but as the years have passed, you've lost touch. You went on with your life, which got busier and more hectic every day, and your abs sort of receded into the background, until you all but forgot about them.

But your abs are still there, hanging out in the old neighborhood, waiting to be found and rediscovered. And eating great food—food that you cook yourself—is the first step in finding them again. Consider:

■ In a study at Penn State, 50 obese subjects were split into two groups. One group ate mostly whole grains—one of the 12 Abs Diet Powerfoods you'll read about in a coming chapter. The other group didn't. After 12 weeks of moderate exercise, both sets of subjects lost weight, but the whole grain group lost mostly belly fat. And their levels of C-reactive protein, an indicator of heart disease and diabetes risk, had dropped by 38 percent.

■ In a study published in the *International Journal of Obesity,* overweight subjects ate 340-calorie breakfasts of either two eggs (another powerfood!) or a bagel 5 days a week for 8 weeks. Those who ate the eggs lost 65 percent more weight than the bagel eaters (and no, their cholesterol levels didn't go up).

■ At Syracuse University, researchers discovered that exercisers who drank high-protein smoothies (yep, it's part of the Abs Diet plan, too) had higher metabolic rates the next day—meaning they burned more fat, even at rest.

■ Simply choosing the right snacks can have a dramatic impact on your weight. The journal *Obesity* recently reported a study showing that people who eat nuts (psst . . . nuts are one of the 12 Abs Diet Powerfoods, too) twice a week are nearly 30 percent less likely to gain weight than people who rarely eat the fiber- and protein-rich snacks.

These studies aren't about cutting calories or spending hours in the gym. They're about the power of eating great food (and more of it!) and how easy it is to trim away belly fat when you know what and how to eat.

My Personal Struggle with Weight

I believe in the power of the Abs Diet because I've seen it work. And I've seen the principles work, not just in my professional life, but in my personal life as well. See, just like most Americans, I, too, have struggled with my weight for years.

As a latchkey kid growing up in the early '80s, I was often left to fend for myself nutritionally. Like most kids, my favorite food group was "beige"—macaroni and cheese, chicken fingers, grilled cheese, and pasta with butter sauce—and I preferred Donkey Kong and the Super Mario Brothers to bikes, balls, and playgrounds. My weight climbed in lockstep with my daily calorie intake and my video game totals, until by age 14 I was hoisting a heifer-like 212 pounds out of bed every morning.

And my weight issues only got worse as I got older: I learned how to drive, which meant that I learned how to drive through. The inherent problem with fast foods is, well, it's fast. When you eat quickly—and I did—the satiety signals your body sends out may register too late, so you consume more calories—and I did—than you would if you ate at a slower pace. With driving, junk food got ever more convenient, and I paid the price for it both with my own embarrassment over my weight and with a constant barrage of humiliation from my older brother, Eric—an elite athlete who was once considered a prospect for the NHL. (The only athletics I got recruited for was the high school wrestling team, where the coach would send me out during tight matches to literally sit on the opposing wrestler in hopes of gaining a draw.)

I felt hopeless. But sometimes, no matter how rough you have it, you realize that others have it rougher. And one person who had it much rougher than me was my father.

My dad was more than 100 pounds overweight for most of his adult life. Over time, he developed hypertension and diabetes, suffered from heart trouble, and would have to stop at the top of a short flight of stairs just to catch his breath. I remember being with him at times, waiting for him to catch his breath, wondering, "Is that what my future will look like?" A massive stroke ended his life at 52. But my father gave me one gift I'll never be able to repay him for: Through his suffering, he showed me what I didn't want to become. Somehow, I had to find a way to turn back the tide of torpid tallow that was surrounding me.

And I got lucky. When I graduated from high school, I joined the Naval Reserve, where the tenets of fitness were gently presented to me in a nurturing, supportive, and convivial atmosphere. (Kidding. They saw a chunky kid from Bethlehem, Pennsylvania, and put him through the wringer, mentally and emotionally. It was the boot camp from hell, but I needed it—and the Navy beat the weight right off me in basic training.)

But just because you can lose weight—especially in an exercise-intensive setting like basic training—doesn't mean you can keep it off when you get older. (Just look at any of those formerly fit NFL players doing play-by-play duty on Sunday afternoon. When forced workouts cease, but the unhealthy eating doesn't, you will gain weight.) What got me truly fit—and what has kept me lean into my early 40s—has been the research I've done as editor-in-chief of *Men's Health*. And that research has led to the nutritional plan that you'll find laid out in these pages.

Why We Need More Abs

To some, the quest for abs might as well be a deep excursion into one's own navel—a vanity exercise for those who are too focused on their self-image. But at a time when more than 130 million Americans are overweight or obese, when one in three children will develop diabetes in adulthood, and when weight-related disease eats up 20 percent of our health care dollars, I'd argue that stripping away inches from your midsection is no quixotic quest. Indeed, it might be the best thing you can do for your health. And the really great news is that it's never too late to get started. Not long ago, a study of 1,600 middle-age adults conducted by researchers at the University of South Carolina revealed that people who began eating five or more fruits and vegetables a day and exercising to keep their weight down reduced their risk of heart disease 35 percent and risk of mortality 40 percent within 4 years of adopting a healthier lifestyle.

The New Abs Diet Cookbook will make it easy for you to lose weight, keep it off, and reap those health benefits. How? By filling you up with powerfoods. The recipes in this cookbook are designed specifically to target belly fat— the most dangerous fat on your body. Belly fat is classified as "visceral fat." That means it is located behind your abdominal wall, where it surrounds your internal organs, pushing your belly outward. And over the past decade, scientists have concluded that the more visceral fat you have, the more it puts your health in danger.

That's because visceral fat doesn't just lie there. It actively works to harm your body by secreting a number of substances, including those called adipokines. Adipokines include a hormone called resistin, which leads to high blood sugar and increases your risk of diabetes; angiotensinogen, a compound that raises blood pressure; and interleukin-6, a chemical associated with arterial inflammation and heart disease. Visceral fat also messes with another important hormone called adiponectin, which regulates the metabolism of lipids and glucose. The more visceral fat you have, the less adiponectin you have and the lower your metabolic rate. (And of course, the lower your metabolism, the easier it is to gain weight—leading to an endless feedback loop of, well, pants with extra belt loops.)

Plus, the more visceral fat you have, the more it may be sabotaging your muscles—leading to even more weight gain, more injury, and less chance of reuniting with your abs. A study in the *Journal of Applied Physiology* showed that those biologically active molecules that are released from visceral fat can actually degrade muscle quality (which again leads to more fat and more health risk). In one study at the University of Alabama–Birmingham, researchers looked at seven different factors that determined a person's heart disease risk. The biggest single predictor of whether you're going to have a heart attack? The amount of visceral fat you're carrying.

Wow. If having abs is a sign of vanity, then it seems like we could sure use a lot more vanity in this country, huh?

So, there's a case for chasing abs. But why do it with a cookbook?

Well, the answer to that one is simple. Most diet plans are about "losing" and "sacrificing." You sacrifice foods you love, the foods that bring enjoyment to your life, in order to lose weight. But who wants to lose? (And who wants to sacrifice foods they love?) How likely are you to be able to swear off barbecued ribs, pizza, spaghetti and meatballs, and all the other foods that many diets ban? That's why diets of denial rarely work after a few weeks or months. We're humans and we like to eat. We don't like sacrifice. Wouldn't you rather gain something and do it while eating great?

I would. That's why *The New Abs Diet Cookbook* brings an entirely new sensibility to the notion of weight control. I don't want you to use this book to lose. I want you to use this book to gain—gain abs, gain muscle, gain control of your weight and your health. And gain a whole new repertoire of healthy meals that you and your family will love! The recipes in the following pages are designed to help you gain all of those things, while effortlessly stripping away fat from your belly and changing your body shape forever.

The Abs Diet focuses on 12 powerfoods that are among the best sources for protein, fiber, and all the other ingredients and nutrients that help your body build muscle and shed fat. It's easy to remember them and work them into your diet by using the acronym ABS DIET POWER: A (almonds and other nuts); B (beans and legumes); S (spinach and other green vegetables); D (dairy—milk, yogurt, cheese); I (instant oatmeal); E (eggs); T (turkey and other lean meats, plus fish); P (peanut butter); O (olive oil); W (whole grains); E (extra-protein (whey) powder); and R (raspberries and other berries). Build your diet around these foods and you'll build a new body in the process. *The New Abs Diet Cookbook* makes that easy for you. Eating the meals detailed in this recipe book in the coming months can help you lose up to 20 pounds of fat (much of it in the first 4 weeks, and from your belly first) and pack on several pounds of lean muscle.

So . . . are you ready to cook up some abs?

The New Abs Diet Cookbook Start-Up Kit

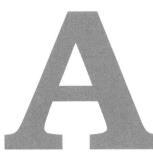

NY JOB IS EASIER when you have the right tools. That's true, too, when the task at hand is cooking healthier foods to stay fit and trim. On the next page, you'll find a handy grocery list containing everything you need to start preparing healthy meals with the Abs Diet Power 12, the nutrient-packed backbone of the New Abs Diet weight-loss program.

You don't have to buy everything at once. Focus your shopping on the Abs Diet Power 12 and expand this list with groceries for specific recipes as needed. At the end of this list, you'll find a selection of cooking tools that'll make your time in the kitchen easier and more efficient.

BASIC TENETS OF THE ABS DIET

NUMBER OF MEALS: Six a day, spaced relatively evenly throughout the day. Eat snacks 2 hours before afternoon and evening meals.

NUTRITIONAL INGREDIENTS TO EMPHASIZE: Protein, monounsaturated and polyunsaturated fats, fiber, calcium.

NUTRITIONAL INGREDIENTS TO LIMIT: Refined carbohydrates (or carbs with a high glycemic load), saturated fats, trans fats, high-fructose corn syrup.

ALCOHOL: Limit yourself to two or three drinks per week to maximize the benefits of the New Abs Diet plan.

ULTIMATE POWERFOOD: Smoothies. The calcium and protein in milk, yogurt, and whey powder—combined with the fiber in oatmeal and fruit—makes them one of the most filling and nutritious foods you can eat (or drink!). You'll find a chapter on smoothies starting on page 91.

THE ABS DIET POWER 12 AND RELATED FOODS

ALMONDS, SLIVERED OR WHOLE, AND OTHER NUTS
Cashews
Pecans
Pistachios
Walnuts

BEANS AND OTHER LEGUMES
Black
Chickpeas (garbanzo)
Kidney
Lentils
Navy
Pinto

SPINACH, FRESH OR FROZEN, AND OTHER GREEN VEGETABLES
Broccoli
Brussels sprouts
Collards
Green or red leaf lettuce
Kale
Romaine lettuce
Spring mix
Swiss chard

DAIRY (FAT-FREE OR LOW-FAT MILK, YOGURT, CHEESES)
Cheddar
Cottage cheese
Feta
Greek yogurt
Monterey Jack
Part-skim mozzarella
Ricotta
Sour cream
Swiss

INSTANT OATMEAL (UNSWEETENED, UNFLAVORED)
Steel-cut oats

EGGS

TURKEY AND OTHER LEAN MEATS
Deli, sliced
Ground
Skinless breasts
Whole

PEANUT BUTTER, ALL-NATURAL (NO ADDED SUGAR)
Almond butter

OLIVE OIL

WHOLE GRAIN BREADS AND CEREALS
Brown rice
Fiber One bran cereal
Spelt
Wheat germ
Whole wheat pasta

EXTRA-PROTEIN (WHEY) POWDER
Chocolate
Vanilla

RASPBERRIES AND OTHER BERRIES, FRESH OR FROZEN
Blackberries
Blueberries
Strawberries

PLUS:

FISH	**FRUIT**	**AVOCADOS**
Clams	Apples	
Halibut	Bananas	**CANNED TUNA**
Scallops	Grapefruit	**VINE & ROOT**
Sea bass	Grapes, red	**VEGETABLES**
Shrimp	Oranges	
Trout	Peaches	**LEAN GROUND**
Wild salmon	Pineapple	**BEEF**

21 TOOLS EVERY COOK NEEDS

We're assuming you have a can opener, a peppermill, and a few serviceable pots and pans. Here are some other helpful items to add to your kitchen quiver if they're not there already.

Avo Saver avocado preserver ($4 gadget keeps cut avocados fresh by reducing exposure to air)

Bamboo cutting boards

Bamboo skewers

Blender

Carrot peeler

Cast-iron skillet

Cedar grill planks

Chef's knife, sharp and well-balanced (we like the Wüsthof Classic 9-inch)

Colander, large

Crock-Pot (slow cooker), 4 quart or larger

Kitchen shears

Knife sharpener

Leatherman Multi-Tool (for cracking nuts, cutting through cans, fixing broken kitchen equipment, and grabbing blue-claw crabs that have escaped)

Meat thermometer

Microplane zester (sure, a kitchen grater will work in a pinch; this will make life easier and tastier)

Salad spinner

Silicone basting brushes

Silicone cooking gloves that reach up to your elbow (much easier to use than tongs for grabbing lobsters out of a pot of hot water or steaks off the back of the grill)

The Way to Cook by Julia Child (a classic handbook of cooking techniques; just beware of the butter)

Waiter's corkscrew

Weber Charcoal Kettle Grill (gas grills are convenient, but nothing beats charcoal)

CHAPTER 1

Find Your Abs in Your Kitchen

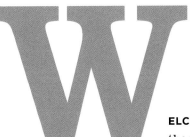

ELCOME TO THE KITCHEN — the room with all the knobs and buttons and stainless steel. You know, where popcorn comes from.

Turn on the light. Look around. Get familiar with this space. You may already be an experienced chef, but if you're like most Americans, cooking isn't your forte. And that's fine, because this isn't a traditional cookbook.

Sure, it's got recipes. And a shopping list. And it's got a lot of phrases like "sauté on high for 3 minutes" and "stir until smooth" and "add a pinch of salt." But that's about as technical as we're going to get. There's nothing exotic or complicated or French in these pages. No, what's in these pages is something even more intriguing: the keys to the body you've always wanted—one with more lean muscle, less flab, and yes, even abs.

That's right. Exercise machines and dumbbells, jump ropes and running shoes may have their place in the pantheon of fitness and weight loss, but the tools in the kitchen are far more powerful than the tools in the gym. Measuring cups and microwaves, sauté pans and soup recipes will become your real fitness buddies, helping you shape up way faster than medicine balls and supersets will.

Your kitchen will help you find your abs, if only by keeping you out of those wastelands of waist expansion: restaurants. A large, 15-year study published in the medical journal *The Lancet* found that people who ate fast food at least twice a week gained an extra 10 pounds a year, compared with those who hit the restaurants less frequently (and, supposedly, made more meals in their kitchens). And the restaurant eaters were twice as likely to develop prediabetes. Other studies show that women and men will consume 200 to 500 more calories per day, respectively, when they eat at restaurants versus when they prepare food at home. That can add up to a pound of fat a week!

Those study results make sense when you consider two facts: One, the obesity rate in this country has doubled since the 1970s; and two, the amount of food dollars we spend on meals made outside the home has also doubled. Those two stats are intrinsically interrelated, because when you turn over the cooking duties to some pimply-faced teen in a paper hat, you lose control over both your ingredients and your portion size. The result: enormous portions, empty calories, bigger waists.

Cooking your meals at home gives you much more control over calories, portion sizes, and exactly what you swallow. I'm a firm believer in the power of food—the right kind of food—to build muscle and burn fat. That's why I've made eating more of the right kinds of foods, more often, a guiding principle of the Abs Diet program.

MORE FOOD = MORE MUSCLE = LESS BELLY FLAB

Make it your mantra, too. It's a brilliantly counterintuitive plan for achieving weight loss, because, hey, who doesn't like to eat?

Not only will you be amazed by the changes you see in your body, you'll also be amazed by how quickly and easily you can whip up filling, nutritious, and truly delectable meals. And there's nothing here that could be confused with rabbit food pellets or "spa cuisine" or the standard "diet" fare. Most of the foods that you'll find here are meaty, gooey, belly filling, and high on the flav-o-meter.

But first, an appetizer: Let's take a look at how your kitchen—and the New Abs Diet nutrition plan—can help uncover that six-pack within you.

FILL YOUR TANK, LOSE YOUR BELLY

New Abs Diet Principle #1: Eat Six Meals a Day

Research reported in the *American Journal of Epidemiology* showed that people who ate smaller meals more frequently—say, four to six times a day—were half as likely to become overweight as people who ate three or fewer times. How does eating more food equal less weight? By maintaining a balance of energy through regular fuel-ups, you keep blood sugar levels stable and control the release of insulin, a hormone that causes the body to hoard fat. That's the scientific explanation, but the plain and simple reason it works is because it does something most diets don't do: It keeps you feeling full, so you won't blow your diet on a binge at the Old Country Buffet.

The exact times on the clock aren't important. What is important is that you eat something containing a mix of carbohydrates, fiber, protein, and a little fat about every 3 hours. Now, how do you do that efficiently? That's where the kitchen comes in. It's your staging area in the battle of the bulge. That's where you plan and prepare your meals and snacks, especially those important ones you take to work. Stock up here and you won't frequent fast-food joints and vending machines for pit stops.

FIRE UP YOUR FAT BURNERS

New Abs Diet Principle #2: Never Skip Breakfast

Cooking (and eating) breakfast starts your day off right by revving up your metabolism, your body's calorie-burning fire. If you skip breakfast, you may reduce your metabolic rate by up to 10 percent, say nutritionists. So, get up 10 minutes earlier and get into the kitchen to make something substantial with oats and eggs, milk and fruit. A recent study from Virginia Commonwealth University showed that a high-protein breakfast (containing 40 grams of protein) can dramatically improve long-term weight loss. In the eight-month study, obese people who regularly ate a 600-calorie breakfast and a small lunch and dinner lost an average of 40 pounds—significantly more weight than people who consumed half the calories for breakfast and just a quarter of the protein. What's more, the big-breakfast eaters kept the weight off much longer. The hormones that transform food into energy prevail at sunrise, so a big breakfast with plenty of protein will speed up your metabolism.

In addition, the protein in eggs, Canadian bacon, milk, and peanut butter will keep you feeling full throughout the morning (so you won't be tempted by

ABS DIET POWER TIP

Here's what your perfect day of strategic eating might look like:

7 A.M.
breakfast

10:30 A.M.
snack

1 P.M.
lunch

3:30 P.M.
snack

6:30 P.M.
dinner

9 P.M.
snack

those Munchkins someone left by the coffeemaker). Protein is satiating and processing protein also boosts calorie burn, say researchers at the University of Illinois. And eating whole grains like oatmeal and barley can make the rest of your meals less fatty. A new Swedish study showed that people who ate barley for breakfast cut their blood sugar response by 44 percent at lunch and 14 percent at dinner, thanks to the high amount of soluble fiber in the grain, which takes hours to digest. And as you learned earlier, the less your sugar and insulin levels spike, the less fat your body will store.

EAT CLEAN, STAY LEAN
New Abs Diet Principle #3: Stick to the Abs Diet Power 12

You'll never know how much fat, sodium, and unpronounceable chemicals are hidden in that fast-food chicken taco salad. But there is one sure way of knowing exactly what you're putting in your mouth: Make your own meals. Your kitchen will never trick you with hidden ingredients as long as you keep your pantry and refrigerator free of most processed and packaged foods. Make a clean sweep of your food supplies. Toss out the sugary cereals, the boxed meals, cookies, crackers, white breads and pastas, fruit-flavored juices, and sodas. Fill your pantry and fridge with the Abs Diet Powerfoods and build your meals and snacks around them. Once again, they are:

ALMONDS AND OTHER NUTS
BEANS AND LEGUMES
SPINACH AND OTHER GREEN VEGETABLES

DAIRY (FAT-FREE OR LOW-FAT MILK, YOGURT, CHEESE)
INSTANT OATMEAL (UNSWEETENED, UNFLAVORED)
EGGS
TURKEY AND OTHER LEAN MEATS

PEANUT BUTTER, ALL-NATURAL (NO ADDED SUGAR)
OLIVE OIL
WHOLE GRAIN BREADS AND CEREALS
EXTRA-PROTEIN (WHEY) POWDER
RASPBERRIES AND OTHER BERRIES

FIGHT CRAVINGS

New Abs Diet Principle #4: Drink Smoothies Regularly

If you don't have a blender with at least 400 watts of ice-chopping power under the hood, go buy one and keep it handy on the kitchen counter. A blender is one of the most effective kitchen gadgets for Abs Diet success. Smoothies made with a mixture of the Abs Diet Powerfoods can act as meal substitutions and hunger-satisfying snacks. These thick, rich, dessertlike concoctions satisfy cravings for sweets, fill your belly with volume, and—when you make them with protein powder—burn fat and build muscle even more effectively. According to a study by British researchers, people who increased the percentage of calories from protein in their meals burned 71 more calories per day than people on low-protein diets. That may not sound like much, but it adds up, to the tune of 7½ pounds lost in a year. Even when the smoothie doesn't call for protein powder, if it's made with milk or yogurt, you'll still reap the muscle-building and weight-control benefits of protein. A 2009 study in the journal *Medicine & Science in Sports and Exercise* showed that women who drank skim milk after exercising lost 3.5 pounds in 12 weeks while another group of women that drank sports drinks actually gained weight.

STOP OVEREATING

New Abs Diet Principle #5: Don't Count Calories

Counting the number of fat grams and calories in a bowl of ice cream is a bummer. Can you think of any better way to lose motivation for healthy eating? Here's a math-free way to keep calories in check: Eat the 12 Abs Diet Powerfoods and their many relatives. The foods themselves will, in a way, count your calories for you. Case in point:

- **EAT 30 STRAWBERRIES** (a powerfood), you get about 70 calories.
- **EAT A SMALL SLICE OF STRAWBERRY CHEESECAKE** (not a powerfood), you get about 320 calories.
- **EAT THE STRAWBERRY SHORTCUT SMOOTHIE ON PAGE 103** (four powerfoods), you get 283 calories plus 14 grams of protein and 5 grams of fiber.

Also, by making your meals in your own kitchen, you wield much more control over another automated calorie-counter: serving size. In 1957, a breakfast muffin weighed 1½ ounces; today, a typical deli or bakery muffin is 8 ounces and 400 calories. Twenty-five years ago, a fast-food cheeseburger contained 333 calories, while today 590 calories is the norm for those enormous sandwiches that pass through the drive-through window. But think about the burgers you cook on your own backyard grill: They're probably closer to the size you ordered while listening to Tears for Fears back in the day. And just think how much saturated fat you can save (up to 23 grams) by making your patties with ground chicken and fiber-rich whole wheat bread crumbs instead of beef. That's something you can't do at the Home of the Whopper.

Here's another reason why making your meals at home will help you lose weight: The dishes in your cabinets aren't the size of manhole covers, as they often are in restaurants. Studies have found a clear correlation between the size of dinner plates and the amount of food people will consume in a sitting. Break out the salad plates when dishing out the spaghetti! And learn to recognize the amount of food in a proper serving size. The Portion-Distortion Decoder on page 13 can help.

SHRINK YOUR BELLY FAT
New Abs Diet Principle #6: Eat More Omega-3s

You've probably heard a lot about omega-3 fatty acids and their link to heart health over the past several years. But did you realize that they are part of the membrane of every cell in your body and they're also the building blocks of hormones that govern many of the functions of organs? The omega-3 fatty acids, particularly EPA and DHA (eicosapentaenoic acid and docosahexaenoic acid, respectively), which you get from cold water fish, may also lower the risk of colon cancer, stroke, asthma, and arthritis and help fight obesity, diabetes, and depression as well. But besides salmon and those smelly little pills they sell at the health food store, what are other ways to get them? You'd be surprised how easy they are to find when you're doing your own shopping and not relying on some fry-cook to scrounge up your meals. The plant-based omega-3, called ALA (alpha-linolenic acid), is found in nuts, whole grains (especially flaxseed), leafy green vegetables, and even in free-range chicken and eggs and grass-fed beef. (The chickens and cows get it from the grass they eat, then pass it on to us. Conventionally raised livestock eat a diet of mostly corn and soy, so they never pick up those healthy omega-3s.) Grass-fed beef also contains more conjugated linoleic acid (CLA), which has been shown to reduce abdominal fat. Focusing on the Abs Diet Power 12 will boost the omega-3 content of your meals like magic. And the delicious seafood recipes you'll find later in this book will have you working more fish dishes into your weekly plan.

STAY TRIM, BEAT DIABETES

New Abs Diet Principle #7: Fight Fat with Fiber

A study at the University of Texas Southwestern Medical Center found that people who boosted their fiber intake from 24 to 50 grams a day enjoyed dramatic improvements in their blood sugar levels. Doctors say the high-fiber diet was as effective as some diabetes medications! Fiber fills us up so we don't overeat. High-fiber foods take longer to chew, which gives your body time to realize that you're no longer hungry, and they digest more slowly, keeping your belly full longer. Fiber slows the release of glucose into your bloodstream, which prevents the blood sugar spikes that can lead to insulin resistance and, eventually, diabetes. Strong epidemiologic data suggests that it helps decrease the risk of coronary heart disease, too.

The American Dietetic Association recommends we consume 20 to 35 grams of fiber per day. Unfortunately, Americans are lucky if they get half that much from the foods they eat. It's even harder to get the most valuable kind of fiber, water-soluble fiber, which binds to cholesterol and ushers it out of the body like a nightclub bouncer.

You're not going to find fiber at the mall food court unless it's in your broccoli, hiding under a sea of Cheez Whiz. Your best strategy for loading up involves stocking your kitchen with high-fiber foods. Don't try to count fiber grams in meals. That'll drive you batty. Rather, simply try to get about 12 servings of a variety of foods, including fruits and vegetables with their skins, beans, lentils and other legumes, nuts and seeds, brown rice, and whole-grain pastas, cereals, and breads. Even snacks can help you get closer to your fiber quota. For example, choose a package of light popcorn instead of a bag of potato chips and you'll get 8 grams of fiber. Wash it down with a low-sodium V8 and you'll gain 2 more.

AVOID EMPTY CALORIES

New Abs Diet Principle #8: Know What to Drink When

I like to drink beer. I like to drink wine and other things, like gin and tonics on hot summer days. But I don't keep six-packs chilling in my refrigerator or open bottles of pinot on the counter for a reason. They are too tempting, too easy to reach for, too full of empty calories.

Are margaritas your cocktail of choice? There are 450 empty calories in that sugar-spiked neon concoction! Alcohol encourages more eating, and it actually causes your body to store fat. When Swiss researchers gave eight healthy men the equivalent in alcohol of about five beers, they found that the alcohol impaired the men's ability to burn fat by 36 percent. Keep your stash of beer and wine somewhere that's a hassle to reach. The basement? A closet? This way, you'll be more likely to limit yourself, as the New Abs Diet advises, to two or three alcoholic beverages a week.

Soft drinks are even a bigger hazard to someone trying to lose weight and belly fat. Sodas and other sugary drinks are the leading source of calories in the average American's diet, accounting for nearly 1 in every 10 calories consumed. On average, every person in the country consumes 52 gallons of soft drinks per year. (That's a lot of sweetness; consider that there are 13 teaspoons of high-fructose corn syrup in just one 12-ounce can of soda.) Soft drinks are particularly problematic because they go down so quickly and effortlessly, and your brain interprets liquids as far less filling than it does solid foods, so it's easy to overconsume. But you can overcome your reliance on soft drinks with a little effort. Put a pitcher of ice water with a slice of lemon in your refrigerator so you'll always have a cold drink at hand. Drink 8 to 12 glasses of the wet stuff a day. Water will help fill you up. It fosters food digestion, helps break down fats and process proteins, and helps keep your metabolism humming. For variety, drink fat-free milk, unsweetened iced tea, and flavored waters. And watch out for fruit juices, seemingly healthful drinks that often pack nearly as much sugar as a can of soda.

STICK TO A HEALTHY EATING PLAN FOR LIFE
New Abs Diet Principle #9: Once a Week, Eat Whatever You Like

Pepperoni pizza? Go ahead. Real buffalo wings? Sure, enjoy! Kung pao chicken with deep-fried egg rolls? Well, okay, if you must. But make it a treat, not a habit.

I want you to ignore all the New Abs Diet principles once a week for an important reason. It will help you to learn control. If you can make it through 6 days of healthy eating and reward yourself for your effort, you'll develop mastery over the human desire for instant gratification. Plus, the food you find in your local restaurant will never compare, in terms of health, nutrition, and flavor, to the foods you're cooking up in your own kitchen. So go ahead, blow your calorie budget on Saturday night by heading out to your favorite restaurant and eating whatever you like. In fact, people who stop going to restaurants and start eating healthier at home often find that their tolerance for sodium changes; restaurant fare is far too salty and actually makes them feel bloated and uncomfortable. It's likely you'll be looking forward to getting back into the kitchen on Sunday.

There's another important reason I encourage you to schedule a cheat day on the New Abs Diet plan. I know that it'll help you change your body. A successful diet plan is about how you eat most of the time, not how you eat all of the time. It's about learning to eat healthier foods, not sacrificing tasty treats for the rest of your life. And a high-calorie day of eating, now and then, can actually help you lose weight by revving up your metabolism. Researchers at the National Institutes of Health found that men who ate twice as many calories in a day as they normally did increased their metabolism by 9 percent in the 24-hour period that followed.

The New Abs Diet has helped so many people lose weight and keep it off because people find it easy to stick with. Unlike other diets that force you to sacrifice the foods you love, the New Abs Diet is a new way of eating that you can adopt for life and actually enjoy more than the way you eat now. Once you try the recipes in this book and see how effectively they strip away belly fat, I know you'll agree.

The New Abs Diet Cheat Sheet (And Portion-Distortion Decoder)

QUARTERBACKS USE wristband crib sheets for play calling all the time. And TV anchors are never far from their blue cards when they're interviewing tough subjects. So, why shouldn't you have a cheat sheet, too?

On the next page you'll find an at-a-glance guide to help you remember the principles of the New Abs Diet peak nutrition and weight-loss plan. We've added a handy portion-distortion decoder to help you recognize proper serving sizes because, you know, we can't tell 3 ounces from 12 either, and even brown rice will weigh you down if you overeat it.

Go ahead and photocopy these two pages (we cleared it with our lawyers). Reduce them by 50 to 75 percent, depending on how good your eyes are. Laminate them if you're ambitious. Put them in your wallet or someplace where you'll be able to use them at restaurants, at work, or while traveling.

THE NEW ABS DIET CHEAT SHEET

■ Eat six meals (including snacks) spaced evenly throughout the day.

■ Plan most meals around the Abs Diet Power 12 food groups.
Each meal should contain at least two of the following:

ALMONDS AND OTHER NUTS

BEANS AND LEGUMES

SPINACH AND OTHER GREEN VEGETABLES

DAIRY (FAT-FREE OR LOW-FAT MILK, YOGURT, CHEESE)

INSTANT OATMEAL (UNSWEETENED, UNFLAVORED)

EGGS

TURKEY AND OTHER LEAN MEATS

PEANUT BUTTER, ALL-NATURAL (NO ADDED SUGAR)

OLIVE OIL

WHOLE GRAIN BREADS AND CEREALS

EXTRA-PROTEIN (WHEY) POWDER

RASPBERRIES AND OTHER BERRIES

■ Emphasize protein, fiber, calcium, and healthy fats
(mono- and polyunsaturated).

■ Limit alcohol (to three drinks per week max); refined carbohydrates
like baked goods, sugar, white bread, rice, and pasta; saturated fats;
trans fats; and high-fructose corn syrup.

■ Cheat once a week by eating anything your heart desires.

■ Exercise for 20 minutes 3 days a week. Two of those strength
workouts should contain abs exercises. On off-workout days,
walk briskly for at least 10 minutes.

THE NEW ABS DIET PORTION-DISTORTION DECODER

Even something as good for you as fish and fruit can add significant calories if you overeat. That's why portion control is an important part of healthy eating. Use this handy guide to help you eyeball a true serving of whatever you eat.

3 ounces lean meat or poultry = deck of playing cards

3 ounces fish = checkbook

1 tablespoon salad dressing = golf ball

1½ ounces hard cheese = 3 stacked dice

1 ounce mozzarella cheese = Ping-Pong ball

1 tablespoon butter or mayonnaise = poker chip

1 cup chili or yogurt = baseball

1 serving popcorn = 3 baseballs

1 baked potato = computer mouse

1 medium fruit = baseball

1 serving almonds = ¼ cup or 12 almonds

1 serving pistachios = ¼ cup or 24 pistachios

1 serving sausage = shotgun shell

1 serving (½ cup) ice cream = tennis ball

4 ounces dried spaghetti = diameter of a quarter when held tightly and viewed from end

½ cup cooked spaghetti = tight fist

8 ounces lasagna = 2 hockey pucks

CHAPTER 2

Introducing the Abs Diet Power 12

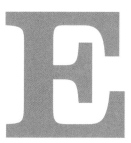

VERY SINGULAR SUCCESS comes from having a great team around you. Face it: Bruce Springsteen would still be looking for an exit off the Jersey Turnpike if it weren't for the guys from E Street. Tom Brady? Just a good-lookin' lug without the Patriots around him. Picking smart teammates is the key to achieving any goal. And the same goes for weight loss.

Well, in this chapter, you're going to meet your team. Get to know them well, trust them, and they'll take care of you for the rest of your life.

If you're new to the Abs Diet, the following pages will explain exactly why the Abs Diet Power 12 food groups are so effective for weight loss. Simply use the acronym—ABS DIET POWER—when you're shopping for groceries, when you're cooking at home, and when you're eating out. And if you're a longtime fan of the Abs Diet, then you already know how effective the power 12 are at stripping away belly fat. In that case, consider this chapter a review, worth reading before digging into the recipes. You'll find surprising new information here based on the latest nutrition science.

Remember, if you build your meals using these 12 powerfoods you won't get involved in a risky guessing game. You'll know exactly what to eat for every breakfast, lunch, dinner, and snack. You'll automatically eat healthier. Here's a quick look at the Abs Diet Power 12 foods and what they'll do for you.

HOW TO READ THE KEY

These icons represent the health benefits of each powerfood.

 BUILDS MUSCLE: Foods rich in muscle-building plant and animal proteins qualify for this seal of approval, as do foods containing certain minerals linked to proper muscle maintenance, such as magnesium.

 HELPS PREVENT WEIGHT GAIN: Foods that fight obesity and reduce your risk of developing diabetes earn this badge. They are typically foods high in fiber and slow-absorbing carbohydrates that keep blood sugar levels stable.

 STRENGTHENS BONE: Calcium and vitamin D are the most important bone builders, and they protect the body against osteoporosis. But beware: High levels of sodium can leach calcium out of bone tissue. Fortunately, all of the powerfoods are naturally low in sodium.

 LOWERS BLOOD PRESSURE: Any food that's not high in sodium can help lower blood pressure—and earn this designation—if it has beneficial amounts of potassium, magnesium, or calcium.

 FIGHTS CANCER: Low-fat, high-fiber diets lower your risk of some types of cancers. New research shows that you can also help foil cancer by eating foods that are high in calcium, beta-carotene, or vitamin C. In addition, all cruciferous (cabbage-type) and allium (onion-type) vegetables get this symbol because research has shown they help prevent certain kinds of cancer.

 IMPROVES IMMUNE FUNCTION: Vitamins A, E, B6, and C; folate; and the mineral zinc help to increase the body's immunity to common illnesses like colds and certain types of disease. This icon indicates a powerfood with high levels of one or more of these nutrients.

 BATTLES HEART DISEASE: Artery-clogging cholesterol can lead to trouble if you eat foods that are predominant in saturated and trans fats, while foods that are high in monounsaturated or polyunsaturated fats will actually help protect your heart by keeping your cholesterol levels in check. The foods wearing this badge also may keep your arteries flexible.

#1: Almonds and Other Nuts and Seeds

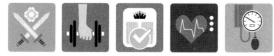

POWER NUTRIENTS: Protein, monounsaturated fats, vitamin E, fiber, magnesium, phosphorus

FIGHTS AGAINST: Obesity, heart disease, muscle loss, wrinkles, cancer, high blood pressure

TRY THESE, TOO: Walnuts, pistachios, peanuts, Brazil nuts, flaxseed, pumpkin seeds, sunflower seeds, and avocados

All nuts are high in protein and monounsaturated fat. But almonds are like Jack Nicholson in *One Flew over the Cuckoo's Nest:* They're the king of the nuts. A 2009 study in the *American Journal of Clinical Nutrition* showed that eating almonds suppresses hunger, and the more you chew them the greater your feelings of fullness will be. In the study, people who chewed 25 to 40 times absorbed more healthy monounsaturated fats and had higher levels of appetite-suppressing hormones than those who chewed just 10 times.

Almonds are nutrient-rich: A handful provides half of the vitamin E you need in a day, 8 percent of the calcium, and 19 percent of your daily requirement of magnesium—a key component for muscle building.

But don't stop at almonds. Walnuts, pistachios, Brazil nuts, and pecans also deliver amazing health benefits. No food packs more selenium than Brazil nuts: 1 ounce has almost 10 times the recommended dietary allowance. University of Arizona scientists recently found that selenium may prevent colon cancer in men. Walnuts, on the other hand, are the only nuts that contain a significant amount of alpha-linolenic acid, the only type of omega-3 fat that you'll find in plant-based food. While you're chomping on walnuts, I want you to consider adding ground flaxseed to your food, which also provides omega-3s, plus 4 grams of fiber per tablespoon. Although not technically a nut, flaxseed has a nutty flavor, so you can sprinkle it into a lot of different recipes, add some to your meat or beans, spoon it over cereal, or add a tablespoon to a smoothie.

WAYS TO EAT MORE:

- **ADD CHOPPED ALMONDS** to plain peanut butter.
- **PUT ALMOND SLIVERS** on cereal, yogurt, or ice cream.
- **FOR A POPCORN ALTERNATIVE,** try the Tailgate Party Nut Mix recipe on page 113.

#2: Beans and Legumes

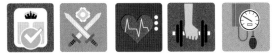

POWER NUTRIENTS: Fiber, protein, iron, folate

FIGHTS AGAINST: Obesity, colon cancer, heart disease, high blood pressure

TRY THESE, TOO: Lentils, peas, bean dips, edamame

Most of us can trace our resistance to beans to some unfortunately timed intestinal upheaval (third-grade math class, a first date gone awry). But beans are, as the song says, good for your heart; the more you eat them, the more you'll be able to control your hunger. In fact, two recent studies found that people who eat a serving of beans daily weigh about 6.6 pounds less, have smaller waist sizes, and have lower blood pressure than people who don't eat beans. Pretty amazing, huh? So, pick your beans: black, navy, lima, pinto, chickpeas (garbanzos)—they're all good (just stay away from refried beans, which are generally made with lard). Beans are a low-calorie food packed with protein, fiber, and iron—ingredients crucial for building muscle and losing weight.

Gastrointestinal disadvantages notwithstanding, beans serve as one of the key members of the Abs Diet cabinet because of all their nutritional power. In fact, you can swap in a bean-heavy dish for a meat-heavy dish a couple of times per week. You'll be lopping a lot of saturated fat out of your diet and replacing it with higher amounts of fiber. Visit page 40 for a list of the best beans, broken down by protein, fiber, and calorie content.

WAYS TO EAT MORE:

- **TOSS INTO SOUPS** and on top of salads.
- **MASH WITH A FORK** and add to burritos.
- **USE HUMMUS** (pureed chickpeas) as a high-fiber substitute for fatty mayonnaise on sandwiches.

#3: Spinach and Other Green Vegetables

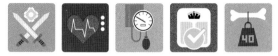

POWER NUTRIENTS: Vitamins, including A, C, and K; folate; minerals, including calcium and magnesium; fiber; beta-carotene

FIGHTS AGAINST: Cancer, heart disease, stroke, obesity, osteoporosis

TRY THESE, TOO: Romaine lettuce; kale; cruciferous vegetables like broccoli and Brussels sprouts; green, yellow, red, and orange vegetables like asparagus, yellow beans, and peppers

You know vegetables are packed with important nutrients, but they're also a critical part of your body-changing diet. I like spinach in particular because one serving supplies nearly a full day's worth of vitamin A and half of your vitamin C. It's also loaded with folate—a vitamin that protects against heart disease, stroke, and colon cancer. Work spinach's mighty cousins, kale and Swiss chard, into your meals, too. Both are loaded with carotenoids, powerful antioxidants that protect your eyes and brain cells from the damage of aging, according to Harvard researchers.

Another potent power vegetable is broccoli. It's high in fiber and more densely packed with vitamins and minerals than almost any other food. For instance, cup for cup, broccoli contains nearly 90 percent of the vitamin C of fresh orange juice and almost half as much calcium as milk. It is also a powerful defender against diseases like cancer, because it increases the enzymes that help detoxify carcinogens. Tip: With broccoli, you can skip the stalks. The florets have three times as much beta-carotene as the stems, and they're also a great source of other antioxidants. You don't have to eat them raw. Steam them and you'll make them even more potent at fighting high cholesterol, researchers at the USDA reported last year.

WAYS TO EAT MORE:

- **PUREE VEGETABLES** and sneak them into marinara sauce or chili.
- **USE SPINACH** as lettuce on a sandwich.
- **STIR-FRY GREENS** with a little fresh olive oil and garlic.

#4: Dairy (Fat-Free or Low-Fat Milk, Yogurt, Cheese)

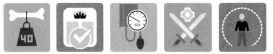

POWER NUTRIENTS: Calcium, vitamins A and B12, riboflavin, phosphorus, potassium

FIGHTS AGAINST: Osteoporosis, obesity, high blood pressure, cancer

TRY THESE, TOO: Cottage cheese, low-fat sour cream

Dairy is nutrition's version of a typecast actor. It gets so much attention for one thing it does well—strengthening bones—that it gets little or no attention for all the other stuff it does well. It's about time for dairy to accept a break-out role as a vehicle for weight loss and muscle growth. Just take a look at the mounting evidence: A University of Tennessee study found that dieters who consumed between 1,200 and 1,300 milligrams of calcium a day lost nearly twice as much weight as dieters getting less calcium. In a Purdue University study of 54 people, those who took in 1,000 milligrams of calcium a day (about 3 cups of fat-free milk) gained less weight over 2 years than those with low-calcium diets. Researchers think that calcium probably prevents weight gain by increasing the breakdown of body fat and hampering its formation.

As for muscle-building, milk is one of the best foods on the planet, because the protein in milk is about 80 percent whey and 20 percent casein. Whey is a terrific protein to consume after your workout, because it is quickly broken down into amino acids and absorbed into the bloodstream. Casein, on the other hand, is digested more slowly, so it provides your body with a steady supply of muscle-building protein for a longer period. Low-fat yogurt, cheeses, and other dairy products can play an important role in your diet. But for your major source of calcium, I recommend milk for one primary reason: volume. Liquids can take up valuable room in your stomach and send the signal to your brain that you're full.

WAYS TO EAT MORE:

■ **USE YOGURT** for low-fat dips.

■ **GRATE HARD CHEESES** on top of your morning oatmeal.

■ **ADD A SPRINKLE OF CHOCOLATE POWDER** to milk to help curb sweet cravings while still providing nutritional power.

#5: Instant Oatmeal (Unsweetened, Unflavored)

POWER NUTRIENTS: Complex carbohydrates and fiber
FIGHTS AGAINST: Heart disease, diabetes, colon cancer, obesity
TRY THESE, TOO: Steel-cut oats and cereals such as All-Bran and Fiber One

Oatmeal is the utility player of your pantry: You can eat it at breakfast to propel you through sluggish mornings, a couple of hours before a workout to feel fully energized, or at night to avoid a late-night binge. I recommend instant oatmeal for its convenience. But I want you to buy the unsweetened, unflavored variety and use other powerfoods such as milk and berries to enhance the taste. Flavored oatmeal often comes loaded with sugar calories.

Oatmeal contains soluble fiber, meaning that it attracts fluid and stays in your stomach longer than insoluble fiber (like vegetables). Soluble fiber is thought to reduce blood cholesterol by binding with digestive acids made from cholesterol and sending them out of your body. When this happens, your liver has to pull cholesterol from your blood to make more digestive acids, and your bad cholesterol levels drop.

Trust me: You need more fiber, both soluble and insoluble. Doctors recommend we get between 25 and 35 grams of fiber per day, but most of us get only half that.

A Penn State study also showed that oatmeal sustains your blood sugar levels longer than many other foods, which keeps your insulin levels stable and ensures you won't be ravenous for the few hours that follow. That's good, because spikes in insulin slow your metabolism and send a signal to the body that it's time to start storing fat. Because oatmeal breaks down slowly in the stomach, it causes less of a spike in insulin levels than foods such as bagels.

Another cool fact about oatmeal: Preliminary studies indicate that oatmeal raises the levels of free testosterone in your body, enhancing your body's ability to build muscle and burn fat, and boosting your sex drive.

WAYS TO EAT MORE:
- **ADD OATS TO MEAT LOAF** in place of bread crumbs.
- **USE HIGH-FIBER CEREALS** to add bulk to yogurt.
- **INCLUDE OATMEAL** in a post-workout smoothie.

#6: **Eggs**

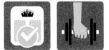

POWER NUTRIENTS: Protein, vitamin B12, vitamin A

FIGHTS AGAINST: Obesity, diabetes, hunger at 10 a.m.

TRY THESE, TOO: Omega-3 eggs and Egg Beaters

For a long time, eggs were considered pure evil, and doctors were more likely to recommend tossing eggs at passing cars than into omelet pans. That's because just two eggs contain enough cholesterol to put you over your daily recommended value. Though you can cut out some of the cholesterol by removing part of the yolk and using the whites, more and more research shows eating an egg or two a day won't end up causing LDL cholesterol or triglyceride levels to rise after all. In fact, a recent study found that people who ate one egg a day for 12 weeks saw their good cholesterol (HDL) levels rise by up to 48 percent. Scientists have recently learned that most bad blood cholesterol is made by the body from dietary fat, not dietary cholesterol. And the niacin found in eggs boosts HDL cholesterol, which helps sweep away bad cholesterol. Rethink your position on eggs and consider taking advantage of this food's powerful makeup of protein. Calorie for calorie, eggs deliver the highest "biological value" of protein—a measure of how well it supports your body's protein need—of any food. In other words, the protein in eggs is more effective in building muscle than protein from other sources, even milk and beef. Eggs also contain vitamin B12, which is necessary for fat breakdown, and taurine, which may reduce the effects of stress chemicals in the brain.

WAYS TO EAT MORE:

▪ **SWIRL AN EGG** into soup to make it more filling.

▪ **ADD A POACHED EGG** to spinach salad and top with shaved Parmesan cheese.

▪ **CRACK AN EGG** and stir it into hot couscous or rice so it cooks right into the grain and adds a creamy texture.

#7: **Turkey and Other Lean Meats**

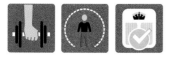

POWER NUTRIENTS: Protein, iron, zinc, creatine (beef), omega-3 fatty acids (fish), vitamins B6 (chicken and fish) and B12, phosphorus, potassium
FIGHTS AGAINST: Obesity, various diseases
TRY THESE, TOO: Lean beef, lamb, fish, shellfish, Canadian bacon

A classic muscle-building nutrient, protein is the base of any solid diet plan. You already know that it takes more energy for your body to digest the protein in meat than it does to digest carbohydrates or fat, so the more protein you eat, the more calories you burn. Many studies support the notion that high-protein diets promote weight loss. In one study, researchers in Denmark found that men who substituted protein for 20 percent of their carbs were able to increase their metabolism and increase the number of calories they burned every day by up to 5 percent.

Among meats, turkey is a rare bird. Turkey breast is one of the leanest meats you'll find, and it packs nearly one-third of your daily requirements of niacin and vitamin B6. Dark meat, if you prefer, has lots of zinc and iron. One caution, though: If you're roasting a whole turkey for a family feast, avoid self-basting birds, which have been injected with fat.

Beef is another classic muscle-building protein. It's the top food source for creatine—the substance your body uses when you lift weights. Beef does have a downside; it contains saturated fats, but some cuts have more than others. Look for rounds and loins (that's code for extra-lean); sirloins and New York strips are less fatty than prime ribs and T-bones. Wash down that steak with a glass of fat-free milk. Research shows that calcium (that magic bullet again!) may reduce the amount of saturated fat your body absorbs.

To cut down on saturated fats even more, replace some of your meat meals with fish dishes and concentrate on cold-water oily fish like tuna and salmon, because they contain a healthy dose of omega-3 fatty acids as well as protein. How important are omega-3s? Well, a 2009 meta-analysis of studies by researchers at the Harvard School of Public Health found that omega-3-deficient diets cause up to 96,000 preventable deaths in the United States each year. The research is clear: We need more fish oil, specifically the omega-3 fatty acids DHA and EPA, in our bodies. Strong evidence from human trials shows that omega-3 fatty acids from fish or fish oil supplements significantly reduce blood triglyceride levels. Fish oil is linked to improvements in blood pressure, prevention of cardiovascular disease, reductions in joint pain from rheumatoid arthritis, and relief from depression, including postpartum depression. And it is now considered a crucial pre-pregnancy supplement for the proper development of the brain. What's more, those fatty acids lower levels of a hormone called leptin in your body, which directly influences your metabolism: The higher your leptin levels, the more readily your body stores calories as fat. Researchers at the University of Wisconsin found that mice with low leptin levels have faster metabolisms and are able to burn fat faster than animals with higher leptin levels. Mayo Clinic researchers studying the diets of two African tribes found that the tribe that ate fish frequently had leptin levels nearly five times lower than the tribe that primarily ate vegetables. A bonus benefit: Several recent population studies report that eating fish regularly or taking fish oil supplements may reduce the risk of developing breast, colon, or prostate cancer.

WAYS TO EAT MORE:

■ **ROLL UP SLICES** of deli turkey breast for a quick protein snack.

■ **INSTEAD OF CANNED TUNA,** have a can of sardines for lunch.

■ **TAKE HIGH-QUALITY FISH OIL** in capsule or liquid form.

#8: Peanut Butter, Natural (No Added Sugar)

POWER NUTRIENTS: Protein, monounsaturated fat, vitamin E, niacin, magnesium

FIGHTS AGAINST: Obesity, muscle loss, wrinkles, cardiovascular disease

TRY THESE, TOO: Almond, cashew, and hazelnut butters

Yes, PB has its disadvantages: It's high in calories, and it doesn't go over well when you try to order it in four-star restaurants. But it's packed with those heart-healthy monounsaturated fats that can help your muscles grow and your fat melt. In one 18-month experiment, people who integrated peanut butter into their diets maintained weight loss better than those on low-fat plans. Also try almond butter. It will provide a bit more fiber and a little less saturated fat, but it blows PB away in the vitamin E department, delivering 40 percent of the RDA versus 14 for PB.

Practically speaking, either butter is a terrific Abs Diet Powerfood because it's a quick and versatile snack, and it tastes good. Since a diet that includes an indulgence like peanut or almond butter doesn't leave you feeling deprived, it's easier to follow and won't make you fall prey to other cravings. Use it on an apple, on the go, or to add flavor to potentially bland smoothies. Two caveats: You can't gorge on it because of its fat content; limit yourself to about 3 tablespoons per day. And you should look for all-natural nut butters, not the mass-produced brands that have added sugar and trans fat.

WAYS TO EAT MORE:

- **DIP PRETZEL LOGS** into peanut butter.
- **FILL CELERY STICKS** with almond butter.
- **MIX 1 TABLESPOON** of peanut butter into plain spaghetti drizzled with soy sauce, sesame seed oil, and Asian vinegar.

#9: Olive Oil

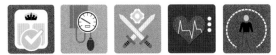

POWER NUTRIENTS: Monounsaturated fat, vitamin E

FIGHTS AGAINST: Obesity, cancer, heart disease, high blood pressure

TRY THESE, TOO: Canola oil, peanut oil, sesame oil

Olive oil and its brethren will help you eat less by controlling your food cravings; they'll also help you burn fat and keep your cholesterol in check. Do you need any more reason to pass the bottle? If so, scan The Oil Business on page 43 to compare these oils with unhealthy fats.

WAYS TO EAT MORE:

▪ **DIP CRUSTY BREAD** into extra-virgin olive oil as an appetizer.

▪ **DRIZZLE OLIVE OIL** and balsamic vinegar on salads instead of creamy bottled dressings.

▪ **SAUTÉ WITH CANOLA OIL** cooking sprays to avoid soaking vegetables and meats in oil.

#10: **Whole Grain Breads and Cereals**

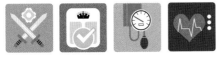

POWER NUTRIENTS: Fiber, protein, thiamin, riboflavin, niacin, pyridoxine, vitamin E, magnesium, zinc, potassium, iron, calcium

FIGHTS AGAINST: Obesity, cancer, high blood pressure, heart disease

TRY THESE, TOO: Brown rice, barley, couscous, quinoa, whole wheat pasta, whole wheat pretzels

When it comes to breads and other things made from cereal grains, here's all you really need to know: Avoid the white stuff.

We're talking about white bread, white rice, and any of those carbohydrates you crave that come in packages and leave your hands greasy: cookies, cakes, buttery Ritz crackers. All those highly processed carbs have had their belly-busting, heart-healthy fiber removed. And you're left with fast-absorbing starches that'll boost and trigger cravings for another bowl of Froot Loops.

Want to know the details? Here's a little biology lesson: Grains like wheat, corn, oats, barley, and rye are seeds that come from grasses, and they're broken into three parts—the endosperm, the germ, and the bran. Think of a kernel of corn. The biggest part of the kernel—the part that blows up when you make popcorn—is the endosperm. Nutritionally, it's pretty much a dud. It contains starch, a little protein, and some B vitamins. The germ is the smallest part of the grain; in the corn kernel, it's that little white seedlike thing. But while it's small, it packs the most nutritional power. It contains protein, oils, and the B vitamins thiamin, riboflavin, niacin, and pyridoxine. It also has vitamin E and the minerals magnesium, zinc, potassium, and iron. The bran is the third part of the grain and the part where all the fiber is stored. It's a coating around the endosperm that contains B vitamins, zinc, calcium, potassium, magnesium, and other minerals.

When food manufacturers process and refine grains, guess which two parts get tossed out? Yup, the bran, where all the fiber and minerals are, and the germ, where all the protein and vitamins are. And what they keep—the nutritionally bankrupt endosperm (that is, starch)—gets made into pasta, bagels, white bread, white rice, and Twinkies.

That's why we say avoid the white stuff. Instead, eat products made with all the parts of the grain—whole grain bread, whole grain pasta, brown rice.

Whole grain carbohydrates can play an important role in a healthy life-style. In an 11-year study of 16,000 middle-age people, researchers at the University of Minnesota found that consuming three daily servings of whole grains can reduce a person's mortality risk over the course of a decade by 23 percent. (Tell that to your buddy who's eating low-carb.) Whole grain bread keeps insulin levels low, which keeps you from storing fat. The Abs Diet and the recipes in this book make strategic use of whole grains, the right kind of carbs, to fill you up, energize your body, and help you lose weight. But don't be fooled by labels that say "wheat bread." It's a trick, a sales ploy to get you to buy something that you think is good for you. Often, it's just made of white flour, devoid of vitamins, minerals, and fiber. Hunt for nutritious products that say "whole wheat" or "whole grain" on the label. Even "multigrain" is a misnomer.

WAYS TO EAT MORE:

- **TRY QUINOA,** a nutty-tasting grain that, like eggs and beef, contains muscle-building amino acids. Use it for pilafs, risottos, or grain salads.

- **USE WHOLE GRAIN BREAD CRUMBS** to reduce the fat content of your meatballs.

- **TURN SALADS INTO BELLY-FILLING MEALS** by adding whole wheat pasta.

#11: Extra-Protein (Whey) Powder

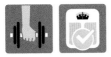

POWER NUTRIENTS: Protein, cysteine, glutathione

FIGHTS AGAINST: Obesity, muscle loss

TRY THIS, TOO: Ricotta cheese

Protein powder? What the heck is that? It's the only Abs Diet Powerfood that you may not be able to find at the supermarket, but it's the one that's worth the trip to a health food store. I'm talking about powdered whey protein, a type of animal protein that packs a muscle-building wallop. If you add whey powder to your meal—in a smoothie, for instance—you may very well have created the most powerful fat-burning meal possible. Whey protein is a high-quality protein that contains essential amino acids that build muscle and burn fat. Researchers at the University of Illinois found that people who eat more protein lose more fat and feel less hungry than people who eat little protein. In their study, subjects who ate more protein were more likely to stick to their diets for 1 year than those who ate more carbohydrates. Whey protein powder is more effective than, say, a steak, because it has the highest amount of protein for the fewest number of calories, making it fat's kryptonite.

WAYS TO EAT MORE:

- **MIX WHEY PROTEIN POWDER** into pancake or cookie batter.
- **STIR INTO COTTAGE CHEESE** or oatmeal.
- **USE ITALIAN RICOTTA.** Made from the whey of cheesemaking, it is lower in fat than cheese, yet high in protein. Ricotta is not just for manicotti. Toss it with pasta or with broccoli and eggs. Mix it with blueberries for a crepe filling. Top a pizza with ricotta.

#12: **Raspberries and Other Berries**

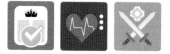

POWER NUTRIENTS: Antioxidants, fiber, vitamin C, tannins (cranberries)
FIGHTS AGAINST: Heart disease, cancer, obesity
TRY THESE, TOO: Blueberries, blackberries, strawberries, raspberries, cranberries, apples, grapefruit, kiwifruit, and most other fruits

Depending on your taste, any berry will do (except Crunch Berries). I like raspberries as much for their power as for their taste. They carry powerful levels of antioxidants, all-purpose compounds that help your body fight heart disease and cancer. The flavonoids in the berries may also help your eyesight, balance, coordination, and short-term memory. One cup of raspberries packs 6 grams of fiber and more than half of your daily requirement of vitamin C. As a general rule, darker and brighter fruits tend to have more vitamins, minerals, and antioxidant compounds. And popular berries like raspberries, blackberries, blueberries, cranberries, and strawberries fall squarely into this category.

Blueberries are particularly strong because they are loaded with the soluble fiber that, like oatmeal, keeps you fuller longer and keeps your blood sugar levels from swinging wildly. Fiber is also a key element in cholesterol control and it can reduce your risk of developing heart disease. Blueberries are all-stars, one of the most healthful foods you can eat. Blueberries beat out 39 other fruits and vegetables in the antioxidant power ratings. (Psst . . . frozen blueberries are just as good for you as the fresh ones. In fact, all fresh berries should be refrigerated to preserve their antioxidants.)

Other fruits, like bananas, kiwifruit, grapes, grapefruit, and oranges, should fill your grocery cart, too. Apples, also known as nature's toothbrush, pack 5,900 cancer-fighting nutrients. How's that for a bargain? And a recent Penn State study demonstrated an apple's potential as a weight-loss tool: People who ate an apple 15 minutes before lunch ended up consuming 187 fewer calories during the meal than those who didn't snack beforehand. The subjects felt fuller afterward, too, thanks to the belly-filling fiber in apples. Apples (as well as grapefruit, strawberries, peaches, and grapes) are rich in a special type of soluble fiber called pectin, which scientists believe may interfere with the body's absorption of cholesterol and may even affect certain enzymes in the liver that produce cholesterol. And all that apple chomping isn't just a good workout for your jaw; it tricks your brain into thinking you're eating more than you really are, say the researchers.

WAYS TO EAT MORE:

- **SLATHER AN APPLE** with natural peanut butter and walk out the door: instant breakfast.
- **DRESS UP AN AVERAGE MAIN DISH** by topping chicken or salmon with strawberries. Stir blueberries into vinaigrette for salads; combine with chopped mangoes for salsa (see Blueberry-Mango Mahi Mahi on page 218).
- **PUREE APPLES** into squash, pumpkin, or cauliflower soups.
- **INSTEAD OF ICE CREAMS,** try fresh berries over vanilla yogurt with chopped peanuts or walnuts. Or dip strawberries in dark chocolate for a delicious one-two antioxidant punch.

CHAPTER 3

Shop (and Cook) Away the Pounds

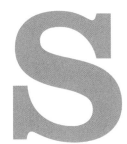

SOME FOLKS JUST LOVE FOOD. They love shopping for food, they love cooking food, they love eating food. They treat food like it's an edible record collection—they absorb trivia like sponges, and they love thinking about it, talking about it, sharing it with others.

Some folks, on the other hand, couldn't care less. Food shopping is a chore, cooking is a pain, and as for the difference between a new potato and an Idaho? Who cares? Food is something to be eaten for fuel, so you can kill those nagging hunger pains and get back to work, play, or watching the tube.

Now, which group do you think is more likely to be overweight: the foodies or the know-nothings?

At first blush, you'd have to assume that the more you love food, the more likely you are to be overweight. But that's exactly wrong: It's the folks who mindlessly scarf down bland fast food while thinking about something else who are more likely to see their weight balloon upward. One study that examined the grocery shopping and eating habits of 1,136 people found that those who looked forward to shopping and employed a strategic approach to food buying by using lists and planning out their week's meals had healthier diets and ate many more whole foods (fresh fruits, vegetables, and grains) than people who felt that food shopping was a chore and employed no particular buying plan. Another study found that those who watched TV during a meal consumed

288 more calories on average than those who focused on what they were eating. And USDA scientists recently studied the eating habits of 1,700 men and women and concluded that the best way to cut calories out of your day was to dine with other people, instead of alone. In other words, the more you focus on your food and the more you share and enjoy it with others, the leaner you'll become.

Isn't it crazy, then, that traditional diet plans make healthy eating seem like a punishment for some ill-defined crime? And that most diet advice boils down to "eat bland food and count calories"? That's exactly wrong: Making food fun is what makes us lose weight. And that, my friends, makes me your kitchen cruise director!

In this chapter, I'm going to show you how to have more fun shopping for, cooking up, and gobbling down great food. And in the process, I'm going to show you how to strip calories off your plate and fat off your belly, just by educating your tastebuds and expanding your kitchen skill set. Consider this: If you learn how to cook portobello mushrooms a few ways and substitute them for beef just once a week, you'll save more than 20,000 calories and about 1,500 grams of fat in a year. That's the equivalent of 5 pounds of weight gone, say researchers at Johns Hopkins Weight Management Center. Replacing low-energy-density foods for high-energy-density ones, even occasionally, they say, is one of the most painless ways to prevent obesity.

Learn more and you'll burn more (calories that is, not the rice). Meal making will go quicker, and you'll have more fun doing it if you can chop vegetables like an Iron Chef and can tell a tenderloin from a rump roast. If you already know all this stuff, our apologies, chef. Jump right into the recipes in the following chapters. But if the kitchen is still terra incognita, consider me your tour guide.

Ready to play?

SHOP RIGHT

Eating well starts with shopping well. If you want to find your abs, fight off injury and disease, and protect your family's well-being—and save a few bucks along the way—you need to learn how to negotiate the supermarket the way Hillary Clinton negotiates a trade agreement. (But without the scowl.) Indeed, when it comes to fitness, the grocery cart is your single most effective tool. Yep, better than dumbbells and a pair of running shoes or a membership at 24-7 Fitness.

Fill that cart with the right foods and you'll be well on your way to losing weight and optimizing your nutrition. Fortunately, you have a head start. You're already armed with a shopping list—the Abs Diet Power 12 and the related foods from the start-up kit. Use it and you gain the advantage over the shopper without a plan.

- **YOU'LL SAVE TIME:** 20 or more minutes than if you shopped by browsing.
- **YOU'LL SAVE MONEY:** $30 or more per visit.
- **YOU'LL SAVE POUNDS** by resisting those seductive whispers emanating from the chips and candy aisles. We've heard 'em, too. It wasn't your imagination.

Don't leave home without your master shopping list. It's essential. So, with said list in hand, here's how to plan your assault on your local supermarket.

NEW ABS DIET SHOPPING TIP #1:
Secure the perimeter.

The folks who design supermarkets have a very specific plan in mind: They want you to spend as much time as possible in the presence of cheap, high-margin junk food. That's why they stick all the fresh, healthy foods along the edges of the grocery store—and why, no matter what supermarket you pop into to buy a carton of milk, you invariably have to walk all the way to the back to find it. (Yeah, sneaky, right?) Get in the habit of working those edges first to load your cart with vegetables, fruits (see Pick Up More Produce, page 45), and meats before easing into the dicey inner aisles. The less time you spend in this belly of the beast, the better.

NEW ABS DIET SHOPPING TIP #2:

Shop on a full stomach.

If you're hungry, you're more likely to reach for a bag of Oreos and start snacking in aisle 7. Everyone knows that. But British scientists studying eating and emotions say that lower serotonin levels in the brain caused by an empty stomach may hamper your willpower. Their research shows that low levels of this brain chemical make it more difficult to control impulsive behavior.

NEW ABS DIET SHOPPING TIP #3:

Keep your head up (and down).

The food marketers know that both kids and adults tend to look at eye level while shopping, so they pay a premium to the supermarkets (called "slotting fees") to have their foods on the middle shelves. What does that mean to you? First, it means that if you buy off the middle shelves, you're paying extra for that real estate, too. Second, it means that the major manufacturers—the ones who make most of the bland, low-nutrient foods on the shelves—rule that lucrative middle ground. The healthier foods tend to be stacked on the top and lower shelves. So, look high and low when stalking the better choices.

NEW ABS DIET SHOPPING TIP #4:

Save trees.

As a general rule, the more packaging a food item requires, the less nutritious it is. The closer you can get to whole foodstuffs, the better. (One exception: frozen fruits and vegetables, which are often packed minutes after picking and can actually be healthier for you.) In general, packaging, processing, and shipping tend to suck the nutrition from food and backfill it with chemical additives. Test yourself: Look in your grocery cart. If more than half of it comes in boxes and bags, you need to reevaluate your diet.

NEW ABS DIET SHOPPING TIP #5:

Hunt for fiber.

When you're buying bread, cereal, or baked goods, look for at least 2 grams of fiber per 100 calories. A bread with 3 to 5 grams per serving will ensure that each sandwich you eat provides 20 to 25 percent of your daily fiber needs. It's worth repeating: We Americans don't get nearly enough of the cholesterol-lowering stuff in a day, typically less than half of the minimum 25 grams recommended by the National Institutes of Health.

NEW ABS DIET SHOPPING TIP #6:
Know how to decode a food label.
Ignore all the confusing extraneous data in tiny type and focus on the important stuff.

- **NUMBER OF INGREDIENTS:** The fewer the better.
- **UNHEALTHY FATS:** If it contains trans fat or if the words "partially hydrogenated" or "interesterified" appear, back away, quickly.
- **SUGARS:** Choose the food with the least amount. Note: Even something as healthy as orange juice can have 20 grams of sugar in an 8-ounce glass.
- **SERVING SIZE OR SERVINGS PER CONTAINER:** This clue will help you avoid overconsuming by accident. A soft drink may list just 80 calories per serving, but the bottle, unbeknownst to you unless you read the nutrition facts label, may contain 2.5 servings. That turns your 80 calories into 200!

NEW ABS DIET SHOPPING TIP #7:
Avoid products with added sugars.
The USDA says the average American consumes 82 grams of added sugars every day. Most comes from soda, baked goods, breakfast cereals, candy, fruit drinks, and sweetened dairy products like yogurt and ice cream. The ingredients list for the product won't help you much if you don't know the many pseudonyms for "sugar," a word that might not even appear on the label. To name a few: high-fructose corn syrup, maltodextrin, barley malt, brown rice syrup, fructose, glucose, lactose, molasses, organic cane juice, sucrose, and turbinado. It's all bad for your body.

NEW ABS DIET SHOPPING TIP #8:
Choose better bread.
Selecting the best sandwich bread takes a bit of recon work. Look for the whole grain bread with the fewest ingredients, suggests David L. Katz, MD, director of the Prevention Research Center at Yale University School of Medicine.

- A whole grain such as wheat, oats, corn, rye, amaranth, or spelt should be the first ingredient listed.
- Don't trust the word *multigrain*. Some breads labeled as such contain two or more refined flours (thus the "multi" moniker) but very little whole grain. Also, ignore those flakes of grain stuck to the bread's crust. Whole grain bread doesn't need to have visible grains.
- The closer you can get to an ingredients list that reads just "whole wheat flour, water, and yeast," the better.
- Check the weight per slice of bread. You can trim your carbohydrate consumption by up to 60 percent simply by choosing loaves whose slices weigh between 15 and 30 grams. Some slices top 45 grams of carbs.

NEW ABS DIET SHOPPING TIP #9:

Avoid flavored yogurts.

They are loaded with sugar. See a pattern here? Pick up the plain yogurts and sweeten them yourself with fresh or dried fruit or a teaspoon of all-fruit-no-sugar jam. Try unflavored Greek yogurt for a change. It has double the protein of regular yogurt and fewer carbohydrates.

NEW ABS DIET SHOPPING TIP #10:

Know your proteins, vegetables, and fats.

As we learned in George Orwell's *Animal Farm*, "All animals are equal, but some animals are more equal than others."

Well, the same goes for fish, nuts, beans, spices, and chile peppers. There's a hierarchy of ingredients for achieving certain culinary goals. And some foods simply have more nutritional value than others. To help guide you as you prepare your shopping list, we offer the following comparison charts for at-a-glance assessment.

CUTS-O'-BEEF DECODER

BOTTOM SIRLOIN: These steaks are somewhat tougher than top sirloin and tenderloin.

BRISKET: From the chest region, it's rippled with fat and can be tough if not marinated. Good for slow-cooked barbecue.

CHUCK: From the muscular shoulder, it's tough but flavorful. Used for ground hamburger and whole for pot roasts.

FLANK: Used for London broil, it's tough with lots of connective tissue but delicious grilled. Slice across the grain.

PLATE: A tough, fatty cut from the front belly. Sold as skirt steak or hanger steak for fajitas or *onglet*, the French bistro steak.

RIB: This is where the rib-eye roasts and steaks come from. This is a well-marbled, tender cut of beef.

ROUND: The large hind leg muscles. Produces rump roast and round rump steak for slow-cooked recipes.

SHANK: Used for soups and stews, this is a tough, sinewy, but flavorful cut.

SHORT LOIN: T-bone and strip steaks and tenderloins, among the most desired cuts.

TENDERLOIN: The most-protected and pampered muscle on the beef, which renders it the most tender and desired. Source of filet mignon and chateaubriand steaks.

TOP SIRLOIN: An excellent grilling steak, more desirable than bottom sirloin.

HOT PEPPER PICKER

	RATING	HEAT LEVEL IN SCOVILLE UNITS
Cherry, Anaheim	1	100–1,000
Cascabel	3	1,500–2,500
Jalapeño, poblano	4	2,500–5,000
Yellow wax, serrano	5	5,000–15,000
Cayenne, Tabasco	7	30,000–50,000
Thai	8	50,000–100,000
Habanero, Scotch bonnet	9	100,000–350,000

FISH FINDER

	TYPE OMEGA-3s (MG EPA & DHA)	PROTEIN(G)	MERCURY LEVEL	ENVIRONMENTAL FRIENDLINESS
Alaskan salmon, wild	923	18	Low	Best
Salmon, farmed	1,671	17	Low	Worst
Mackerel	1,700	16	Low	Good
Herring	1,900	12	Low	Best
Trout, farmed	789	18	Low	Best
Halibut	308	18	Medium	Best
Yellowfin tuna	185	20	Medium	Good
Mahi mahi	92	16	Medium	Good
Swordfish	543	17	High	Good
Grouper	210	16	Medium	Varies
Tilapia	102	17	Low	Best
Sardines	500	22.7	Low	Best
Catfish, farmed	233	13	Low	Best
Atlantic cod	156	15	Low	Varies
Chilean sea bass	506	16	Medium	Worst

All values are per 3 ounces.

BEAN COUNTER

	FIBER (G)	PROTEIN (G)	ANTIOXIDANTS (MMOL)	CALORIES
Black beans[1]	8.7	8.9	8,040	132
Chickpeas (garbanzos)[2]	7.6	8.9	847	164
Green beans[3]	3.2	1.9	759	35
Navy beans[4]	10.5	8.2	1,520	140
Pinto beans[5]	9	9	7,779	143
Red kidney beans[6]	7.4	8.7	8,459	127

All values are per 100 grams cooked.

BENEFITS

[1] Top in cancer-fighting chemicals, according to Cornell researchers.

[2] May reduce levels of the hormone insulin, lowering your risk of diabetes.

[3] May lower homocysteine, which has been linked to vascular disease.

[4] High in folate, a B vitamin that may prevent stroke and cognitive decline.

[5] An Arizona State study found that eating ½ cup a day can slash LDL cholesterol by 9 percent.

[6] One of the richest bean sources of antioxidants that may help prevent hardening of the arteries.

ABS DIET POWER TIP

Choose dried over canned beans to reduce sodium. Soak them overnight to hydrate. No time to soak? Then rinse and drain your canned beans before adding them to recipes.

MEAT O'MATIC

Pork or turkey? Beef or bison? The chart below arranges different animals and cuts of meat on the same playing field so you can choose the healthiest fare without having to research fat grams and beneficial nutrients. We've calculated it all for you: By assigning point values to protein-to-fat ratio, nutrient density, and fat and cholesterol content, we're able to consider pork loin versus porterhouse steak for dinner tonight.

HOW TO READ THE SCORE:
The higher the number, the more nutritious the meat.

   6+ means eat regularly

   4–5.99, eat occasionally

   0–3.99, eat rarely

BEEF

Round	4.91
Flank	4.73
Top loin	4.25
Ground, grass fed	4.13
T-bone	3.92
Top sirloin	3.90
Ground, 90% lean	3.87
Tongue	3.77
Porterhouse	3.75
Brisket, whole	3.71
Rib eye, small end	3.60
Tenderloin	3.45
Ground, 80% lean	3.38
Rib roast, whole	3.20

BISON

Top sirloin	6.75
Ground, grass fed	4.63

CHICKEN

Light meat	7.38
Dark meat	5.99
Giblets	5.97

DUCK

Breast	5.22
Leg	3.90

LAMB

Shoulder	4.21
Ground	3.15

OSTRICH

Top loin	7.09
Ground	5.64

PORK

Tenderloin	6.90
Top loin/loin chops	5.92
Center loin/center rib	5.39
Sirloin	5.13
Ribs	4.72
Spareribs	4.09
Blade chops/roast	4.02
Ham, whole	3.24
Bacon, cured	3.03

TURKEY

Light meat	7.34
Dark meat	5.55
Ground	4.71

NUT CRACKER

Nuts are rich in the artery-clearing tag team of fiber and monounsaturated fat. To get the heart benefits without gaining weight, eat a handful of one type daily, plus two Brazil nuts for cancer protection.

	FIBER (G)	PROTEIN (G)	MONOUNSATURATED FAT (G)	EXTRAS
Almonds	3	6	8.6	7.3 mg vitamin E
Brazil nuts	2	4	7	544 mcg selenium
Cashews	1	5	6.7	82 mg magnesium
Hazelnuts	3	4	12	27 mg phytosterols
Peanuts	2	7	6.8	67.2 mcg folate
Pecans	3	3	12	144 mmol antioxidants
Pine nuts	3	3	6.4	1.2 mg manganese
Pistachios	3	6	7	61 mg phytosterols
Walnuts	2	4	2.5	2.5 g omega-3s

All values are per 1 ounce.

SPICE ROUTE

Sprinkle your food with free-radical fighters.

	ANTIOXIDANT CAPACITY (MMOL PER KG)		ANTIOXIDANT CAPACITY (MMOL PER KG)
Saffron	53	Oregano	30.7
Bay leaf	47.9	Thyme	30.5
Rosemary	44	Sage	23.4
Paprika	40	Basil	21.8
Black pepper	37	Mint	8.8

THE OIL BUSINESS

Choose the healthiest fats and the right ones for the job. (All values are per 1 tablespoon.)

CANOLA OIL Calories: 124

Saturated fat: 0.9 g — Monounsaturated fat: 8.2 g

Polyunsaturated fat: 4 g — Trans fat: 0 g

USE FOR: Stir-fries, eggs, most any kind of frying since it stands up to high heat.

PEANUT OIL Calories: 119

Saturated fat: 2.3 g — Monounsaturated fat: 6.2 g

Polyunsaturated fat: 4.3 g — Trans fat: 0 g

USE FOR: Wok or deep-frying because of its high smoke point.

OLIVE OIL Calories: 119

Saturated fat: 1.8 g — Monounsaturated fat: 10 g

Polyunsaturated fat: 1.2 g — Trans fat: 0 g

USE FOR: Vegetables and salads, because it's more flavorful than canola oil. For high-heat cooking, choose a variety other than extra-virgin. Virgin and light olive oils both have higher smoke points, so they can withstand more heat without imparting bitter flavors and potentially toxic substances.

SESAME OIL Calories: 120

Saturated fat: 1.9 g — Monounsaturated fat: 5.4 g

Polyunsaturated fat: 5.1 g — Trans fat: 0 g

USE FOR: The darker, toasted style of sesame oil is used as a condiment in sauces, noodles, and stir-fries after cooking.

SOYBEAN OIL Calories: 120

Saturated fat: 2 g — Monounsaturated fat: 5.4 g

Polyunsaturated fat: 5.6 g — Trans fat: 0 g

USE FOR: Don't bother. There are healthier oils to use than this cheap stuff.

LARD Calories: 115

Saturated fat: 5 g —————————— Monounsaturated fat: 5.8 g

Polyunsaturated fat: 1.4 g —————————— Trans fat: 0 g

USE FOR: Baked goods instead of butter, because it has fewer artery-clogging saturated fats. Limit consumption.

BUTTER Calories: 102

Saturated fat: 7.2 g —————————— Monounsaturated fat: 3.3 g

Polyunsaturated fat: 0.5 g —————————— Trans fat: 0 g

USE FOR: Pastries, cakes, and other baked goods for creamier, melt-in-your-mouth desserts.

TIP: For spreading on toast or vegetables, use whipped butter, which has half the fat and calories of regular butter.

MARGARINE Calories: 100

Saturated fat: 1.6 g —————————— Monounsaturated fat: 4.2 g

Polyunsaturated fat: 2.4 g —————————— Trans fat: 3 g

USE FOR: Don't. Hydrogenation, the manufacturing process that turned the liquid vegetable oil into a solid fat, created dangerous trans fat. Coloring and artificial flavors have also been added to help this man-made concoction look more like natural butter.

PICK UP MORE PRODUCE

We've seen your future, and it includes parsnips.

When you learn that one serving of this sweet root vegetable packs twice the fiber of a sweet potato and oodles of blood-pressure-lowering potassium and vitamin C, we think you'll be more inclined to try one—maybe baked with a little olive oil. What do you think?

Knowing your produce and how to prepare it is a key step toward getting more fruits and vegetables into your diet. And, God knows, we can all benefit from spending more time in the produce department. A large-scale Harvard study found that people who consumed eight or more servings of fruits and vegetables a day were 30 percent less likely to have a heart attack or stroke than those who ate less than 1½ servings a day. That's a significant preventive measure. What's more, eating more whole produce is one of the easiest ways to lose weight. In one study, people who ate an apple appetizer before dinner consumed 187 fewer calories by the end of the meal than those who didn't eat the fiber-rich snack. Other new research shows that eating an apple a day lowers risk of prediabetes by 27 percent.

Now, maybe you're thinking: apples? You're sick of apples. And parsnips are too, um, Eastern European for your palate. Well, that's fine because there are many more options to choose from that'll pay off with similar benefits. Just look at them all . . .

ARTICHOKES

What's inside: A higher total antioxidant capacity than any other common vegetable, according to USDA tests.
Look for: Deep green, tightly closed leaves. The leaves should squeak when pinched together.
How to store: In the fridge in a plastic bag for up to 5 days.

ARUGULA

What's inside: Vitamin K, which may improve insulin sensitivity, offering protection against diabetes.
Look for: Emerald green leaves that are not yellowing or limp. The smaller the leaf, the less pungent its bite.
How to store: In the fridge in a plastic bag for up to 3 days.

ASPARAGUS

What's inside: Folate, a B vitamin that protects the heart by helping to reduce inflammation.

Look for: Vibrant green spears with tight purple-tinged buds. Thinner spears are sweeter and more tender.

How to store: Trim the woody ends and stand the stalks upright in a small amount of water in a tall container. Cover the tops with a plastic bag and cook within a few days.

AVOCADOS

What's inside: Plenty of cholesterol-lowering monounsaturated fat.

Look for: Firm flesh. Avoid avocados with sunken, mushy spots. They should not rattle when shaken—a sign the pit has pulled away from the flesh.

How to store: To ripen, place avocados in a paper bag and store at room temperature for 2 to 4 days. To speed up this process, add to the bag an apple, which emits ripening ethylene gas. Place ripe avocados in the fridge for up to 1 week.

BANANAS

What's inside: Vitamin B6, which helps prevent cognitive decline, according to scientists at the USDA.

Look for: Ripe bananas have uniform yellow skins or small brown freckles, indicating they are at their sweetest. Avoid any with evident bruising or split skins.

How to store: Keep unripe bananas on the counter, away from direct heat and sunlight (speed things up by placing green bananas in an open paper bag). Once ripened, refrigerate; though the peel turns brown, the flavor and quality are unaffected.

BEETS

What's inside: Nitrate, which may help lower blood pressure.

Look for: Smooth, deep-red surface that's unyielding when pressed. Smaller roots are sweeter and more tender. Attached greens should be deep green and not withered.

How to store: Remove the leaves (which are great sautéed in olive oil) and store them in a plastic bag in the fridge for no more than 2 days. The beets will last in the crisper for up to 2 weeks.

BELL PEPPERS

What's inside: All bell peppers are loaded with antioxidants, especially vitamin C. Red peppers lead the pack, with nearly three times the amount of vitamin C found in fresh oranges. A single serving also has a full day's worth of vision-protecting vitamin A.

Look for: Lively green stems. Lots of heft for their size, with a brightly colored, wrinkle-free exterior.

How to store: Refrigerate in the crisper for up to 2 weeks.

CABBAGE

What's inside: More than half your vitamin K requirement in just 1 cup.

Look for: Tightly packed, crisp, deeply hued leaves free of blemishes. Should feel dense when lifted; it's best that the stem not have any cracks at its base.

How to store: Tightly enclose cabbage in a plastic bag and store in the fridge for up to 10 days.

CANTALOUPE

What's inside: Loads of vitamin C, which may offer protection against having a stroke.

Look for: The stem end should have a smooth indentation. Look for a sweet aroma, slightly oval shape, and a good coverage of netting. The blossom end should give slightly to pressure. Avoid those with soft spots—an indication of an overripe melon.

How to store: Ripe cantaloupes should be stored in plastic in the fridge for up to 5 days, after which they begin to lose flavor.

CARROTS

What's inside: Beta-carotene, the source of vitamin A, which helps fight off infections.

Look for: Smooth and firm with bright orange color. Avoid those that are bendable or cracked at the base. Bunches with bright green tops still in place are your freshest choice.

How to store: Store carrots in the crisper in a plastic bag with the greens removed for up to 3 weeks.

CAULIFLOWER

What's inside: Detoxifying compounds called isothiocyanates, which offer protection against some forms of cancer.

Look for: Ivory white and compact florets with no dark spotting on them or the leaves. The leaves should be verdant and firm.

How to store: Refrigerate, unwashed, in a plastic bag for up to 1 week. If light brown spots develop on the florets, shave off with a paring knife before cooking.

CELERY

What's inside: Luteolin, a flavonoid linked to reduced brain inflammation, a risk factor for Alzheimer's.

Look for: Solid, tight stalks with only a few, if any, cracks, and vivid green, not yellowing, leaves. The darker the celery, the stronger the flavor.

How to store: Sturdy celery can be stored in the fridge in a plastic bag for 2 weeks.

EGGPLANT

What's inside: Chlorogenic acid, a phenol antioxidant that scavenges disease-causing free radicals.

Look for: Good weight to them with tight, shiny, wrinkle-free skin. When they're pressed, look for them to be springy, not spongy. The stem and cap should be forest green, not browning.

How to store: Store eggplants in a cool location (not the fridge) for 3 to 5 days. Eggplants are quite sensitive to the cold.

FIGS

What's inside: Phytosterols, which help keep cholesterol levels in check.

Look for: Plump with deeply rich color; soft but not mushy to the touch. Avoid those with bruises or a sour odor.

How to store: Place fresh figs on a plate lined with a paper towel and eat them as they ripen. They bruise easily, so gentle handling is prudent. They also ripen quickly, so eat within a few days of purchasing. If overripe, simmer with a bit of water, sugar, and balsamic vinegar for a fig jam or sauce.

GARLIC

What's inside: The cancer-fighting compound allicin, that can also cut down Helicobacter pylori—bacteria responsible for the development of stomach ulcers.

Look for: The bulb should feel heavy for its size, with tightly closed cloves in the bulb that remain firm when gently pressed. The skin can be pure white or have purple-tinged stripes and should be tight fitting.

How to store: Place bulbs in a cool, dark, well-ventilated location for up to 1 month.

GRAPEFRUIT

What's inside: Anticancer lycopene and 120 percent of daily vitamin C needs in 1 cup.

Look for: A heavy fruit (a sign of juiciness) with thin skin that is a tad responsive to a squeeze. Small imperfections in color and skin surface are not detrimental to the sweet-tart flavor. Yet, avoid any that are very rough or have soft spots. The same criteria apply for oranges.

How to store: Refrigerate for up to 3 weeks.

GRAPES

What's inside: Resveratrol, a potent antioxidant in red and purple grapes that offers protection against cardiovascular disease.

Look for: Plump, wrinkle free, and firmly attached to the stems. There should be no browning at the stem connection, but a silvery white powder ("bloom") keeps grapes, especially darker ones, fresher longer. Red grapes are best if full-colored with no green tinge. Green grapes with a yellowish hue are the ripest and sweetest.

How to store: Loosely store, unwashed, in a shallow bowl in the fridge for up to 1 week.

GREEN BEANS

What's inside: Fiber (4 grams in 1 cup cooked), which can reduce disease-related mortality, according to Dutch researchers.

Look for: Vibrant, smooth surface without any visible withering. They should "snap" when gently bent.

How to store: Refrigerate, unwashed, in an unsealed bag for up to 1 week.

KALE

What's inside: Lutein, an antioxidant in the retina that protects against vision loss.

Look for: Dark blue-green color with moist leaves. The smaller the leaves, the more tender the kale. Avoid wilted foliage with discolored spots.

How to store: Peppery kale is best kept in the fridge tightly wrapped in a plastic bag pierced for aeration, where it will last 3 to 4 days.

KIWI

What's inside: Only 56 calories for a large one and 20 percent more of the antioxidant vitamin C than an orange.

Look for: Softness, but not too much give. Steer clear of those that are mushy, wrinkled, or bruised with an "off" smell.

How to store: Keep at room temperature to ripen. To quicken the process, place in a paper bag with an apple. Once ripened, place in the fridge in a plastic bag for up to 1 week.

LEEKS

What's inside: Good amounts of eye-protecting lutein, manganese, and vitamins A, C, and K.

Look for: Green, crisp tops with an unblemished white root end. Gravitate toward small to medium leeks, which are less woody and tough than larger ones. Those with spotted or yellowing leaves should be ignored.

How to store: Loosely wrapped in plastic in the fridge, they'll keep fresh for a week.

LEMONS/LIMES

What's inside: Phytonutrient liminoids, which appear to have anticancer, antiviral properties.

Look for: Brightly colored fruit that's well-shaped with smooth, thin skin. They should feel sturdy but give ever so slightly when squeezed. Small brown splotches on limes do not affect flavor (although they are a sign of deterioration, and those with splotches should be consumed first).

How to store: At room temperature, in a dark location, for about 1 week or refrigerate for up to 2 weeks.

LETTUCE: RED LEAF, GREEN LEAF, OR ROMAINE

What's inside: Vitamin K, which is needed for blood clotting and bone health.

Look for: Crisp romaine leaves that are free of browning edges and rust spots. The interior leaves are paler in color with more delicate flavor. Avoid red and green leaf lettuce with signs of wilting.

How to store: Refrigerate for 5 to 7 days in a plastic bag.

MANGOES

What's inside: A good showing of vitamins A, B6, and C, plus fiber.

Look for: Mangoes to be eaten shortly after purchase should have red skin

with splotches of yellow, and the soft flesh should give with gentle pressure. Mangoes for later use will be firmer with a tight skin, duller color, and green near the stem.
How to store: Ripen at room temperature until fragrant and giving. Ripe mangoes can be stored in the fridge for up to 5 days.

MUSHROOMS: BUTTON, CREMINI

What's inside: Immune-boosting, tumor-suppressing complex-carbohydrate polysaccharides.
Look for: Tightly closed, firm caps that are not slimy or riddled with dark soft spots. Open caps with visible gills indicate consumption should be a priority.
How to store: Place meaty mushrooms on a flat surface, cover with a damp paper towel, and refrigerate for 3 to 5 days.

ONIONS

What's inside: GPCS, a peptide shown to reduce bone loss in rats, plus the cancer-fighting compound quercetin.
Look for: Nice shape with no swelling at the neck and dry, crisp outer skin. Lackluster onions have soft spots, green sprouts, or dark patches.
How to store: Keep onions in a cool, dark location away from potatoes for 3 to 4 weeks.

PAPAYAS

What's inside: A complete nutritional package, including plenty of fiber and vitamins C, A, E, and K.
Look for: Beginning to turn yellow and somewhat-yielding flesh when lightly squeezed. Avoid papayas that are awash in green, have dark spots, or are shriveled. Blotchy papayas often have the most flavor.
How to store: Once ripe, eat immediately or refrigerate for up to 3 days. Unripe, greener papayas should be ripened at room temperature in a dark setting until yellow blotches appear.

PEACHES

What's inside: Vitamin C, antioxidant beta-carotene, fiber, and potassium.
Look for: Fruity aroma with a background color that is yellow or a warm cream color. Those destined for immediate consumption yield to gentle pressure along their seams without being too soft. For future intake, opt for those that are firm but not rock hard. Red blush on their cheeks is variety dependent

and is not a ripeness indicator.

How to store: Store unripe peaches at room temperature open to air. Once ripe, toss into the refrigerator and consume within 2 to 3 days.

PEARS

What's inside: Belly-busting fiber and vitamin C—as long as you eat them with the skin on.

Look for: Pleasant fragrance with some softness at the stem end. The skin should be free of bruises, but some brown discoloration (russeting) is fine. Firmer pears are preferable for cooking use.

How to store: Ripen at room temperature in a loosely closed brown paper bag. Refrigerate once they're ripe and consume within a couple of days.

PINEAPPLE

What's inside: Bromelain, an enzyme with potent anti-inflammatory powers and blood-thinning properties. It's used to treat arthritis.

Look for: Vibrant green leaves with a bit of softness and a sweet fragrant aroma from the stem end. Avoid spongy fruit with brown leaves or a fermented odor.

How to store: Keep a pineapple with a weak aroma at room temperature for 2 to 3 days until it softens slightly. Then refrigerate for up to 5 days.

POMEGRANATES

What's inside: Hefty amounts of antioxidants shown to improve sperm quality, thus boosting fertility.

Look for: Pick pomegranates that are weighty for their size with glossy, taut, uncracked skin that is deep red. Gently press the crown end—if a powdery cloud emanates, the fruit is past its prime.

How to store: Stored in a cool, dry location, pomegranates keep fresh for several weeks (up to 2 months in the fridge).

POTATOES: SWEET, WHITE

What's inside: Potassium, which may help preserve muscle mass as we age.

Look for: Unyielding, with smooth undamaged skin. Avoid if bruised, cracked, or green tinged. Loose spuds tend to be better quality than bagged.

How to store: Outside of the fridge, in a cool, dark place separated from onions, potatoes will last for months. Sweet potatoes, however, should be used within a week.

RASPBERRIES

What's inside: More fiber (8 grams per cup) than any other commonly consumed berry, plus the anticancer chemical ellagic acid.

Look for: Plump and dry berries, with good shape and intense, uniform color. Examine the container carefully for mold or juice stains at the bottom. Raspberries with hulls attached are a sign of an underripe, overly tart berry.

How to store: Place highly perishable raspberries, unwashed, on a paper towel in a single layer. Cover with a damp paper towel and refrigerate for no more than 2 to 3 days.

SPINACH

What's inside: Chromium, which is involved in carbohydrate and fat metabolism and may reduce hunger and food intake.

Look for: Opt for bunches with leaves that are crisp and verdant green, with no spots, yellowing, or limpness. Thin stems are best, as thick ones are a sign of more bitter, overgrown leaves.

How to store: Pack unwashed spinach bunches loosely in plastic bags and store in the fridge for 3 to 4 days.

STRAWBERRIES

What's inside: The most vitamin C of any of the commonly consumed berries.

Look for: Seek out unblemished berries where the bright red color extends all the way to the stem. Good berries should have a strong fruity smell and be neither soft and mushy nor hard and firm. Smaller strawberries often have more flavor than the oversized megamart versions.

How to store: Place unwashed strawberries in a single layer on a paper towel in a covered container. They will last for 2 to 3 days in the fridge.

TOMATOES

What's inside: Lycopene, a carotenoid antioxidant that helps fend off certain cancers.

Look for: Go only for heavy tomatoes that are rich in color and free of wrinkles, cracks, bruises, or soft spots. They should have some give, unlike the rock-solid ones bred for transport. Too soft, though, and the tomato is likely overripe and watery. Off-season, select more flavorful smaller versions like plum (Roma) and cherry tomatoes.

How to store: Never store tomatoes in the fridge; the cool temps destroy flavor and texture. Keep them at room temperature out of direct sunlight for up to 1 week.

WATERMELON

What's inside: Citrulline, an amino acid that's converted to arginine, which relaxes blood vessels, thus improving blood flow.

Look for: Dense, symmetrical melons that are free of cuts and sunken areas. The rind should appear dull, not shiny, with a rounded creamy-yellow under- side that shows where ground ripening took place. A slap should produce a hollow thump.

How to store: Store whole in the fridge for up to 1 week. The cold prevents the flesh from drying out and turning fibrous.

ZUCCHINI

What's inside: Riboflavin, a B vitamin needed for red blood cell production and for converting carbohydrates to energy.

Look for: Purchase heavy, tender zucchini with unblemished deep green skins that are adorned with faint gold specks or strips. Smaller zucchini are sweeter and more flavorful.

How to store: Refrigerate in the crisper in a plastic bag for up to 5 days.

HOW TO COOK LIKE
THE NEXT FOOD NETWORK STAR

If you can put together an office desk from IKEA, you can cook a tasty, nutritious meal for yourself and your family. It's just a matter of following directions, and (what luck!) the back half of this book is loaded with them—simple recipes for good food.

Don't fear the fire pit (or the microwave).

A baboon can grill a steak. Making great meals is more about assembling the best ingredients in the right quantities than wielding utensils like a hibachi chef. Learn a few tricks, however, and you'll have more fun even before you sit down to eat.

Master slow-cooking.

Owning a Crock-Pot is better than having a live-in chef. The meal cooks while you're at work, and you don't have to worry about anyone raiding your wine fridge. Slow-cooking is a nearly fail-proof way to make flavorful low-fat meals without previous experience. If you can fill a pot with meat and vegetables, you're hired. A couple of things to know before you go slow: You can't go wrong with a 6-quart Crock-Pot. It's the perfect size for a family, and if it's just you, well, you can always freeze the leftovers. Tougher cuts of meat, like stew beef, are perfect for the slow cooker. Cut them into chunks and toss into the bottom of the pot before adding vegetables. They'll be fork tender by dinnertime.

Master poaching fish.

I've always grilled or broiled my catch, even when catching it meant snagging a fillet out of the ice at my fish market. Then a nutritionist/chef friend of mine turned me on to a wonderfully simple way of cooking my favorite salmon (or bass, cod, or halibut) without adding fat: poaching. And the blessing of poaching is that it's almost impossible to overcook the fish. How to do it:

1. **FILL A SAUTÉ PAN** with about an inch of water; toss in a few cloves of garlic, about 20 peppercorns, some parsley sprigs, a bay leaf, and maybe a cut-up carrot or two.
2. **COVER THE SAUCEPAN** and allow the mixture to come to a boil. Turn down

the heat to low. No more boiling. Let the poaching liquid simmer for about 15 minutes so the spices infuse the water. Then, using a slotted spatula, place the fish fillets into the broth bath. Cover for about 5 minutes (longer for thicker fillets).

3. **REMOVE THE FISH** from the liquid and top with just a bit of extra-virgin olive oil, a squeeze of lemon, kosher salt, and a few drained capers. Nothing more. Poaching is the healthiest form of fish cooking because the flavor of the fish is not overwhelmed by sauces or marinades.

Master stir-frying.

Here's what I love about stir-frying: easy cleanup. You've got one pot. The entire meal goes from wok to plate. Another plus: It's low-fat cooking at its fastest, especially if you buy precut vegetables and protein. Sometimes, when I'm crunched, I hit the salad bar at the deli to pick a container of cut, ready-to-go vegetables—including a tong's worth of those Chinese baby corns. Then it's just a matter of choosing protein and turning up the heat. Wok this way . . .

1. **START WITH HIGH HEAT** and add just enough olive or canola oil to coat the wok, about 2 tablespoons. When the oil is hot (but not smoking hot), add the chopped protein and cook it until it changes color, mixing it constantly with a wooden spoon to ensure even cooking. Remove the meat, fish, or poultry and set aside.

2. **SCRUB THE WOK QUICKLY** under cold water to wash out any protein bits that might burn and taint the flavor of your vegetables. Return the wok to the heat and coat with new oil. When hot, add a teaspoon of garlic and cook for 15 seconds.

3. **ADD EVENLY CUT VEGETABLES** and cook for 2 minutes. Keep moving them around with your wooden spoon to cook evenly. A perfectly stir-fried vegetable is fork-tender with a little crunch. Add a splash of Chinese cooking wine and let everything sizzle for a few seconds.

4. **ADD BACK THE PROTEIN** to the wok. Many Chinese chefs add $\frac{1}{3}$ cup broth and a pinch of cornstarch. Cook over high heat until the broth thickens, about 1 minute, then add a few shakes of soy sauce.

Master grilling.

Choose your fire. Charcoal grills make for tastier meats, but propane grills are generally healthier for cooking. One study found that charcoal-grilled meats contained more carcinogens called polycyclic aromatic hydrocarbons (PAHs) than meat heated with propane-fueled flames. When fat drips from the meat and burns, it creates PAH-infused smoke, which coats what you're cooking. Charcoal, by nature, creates more smoke than gas does. Not only that, it burns hotter, which chars meat and creates heterocyclic amines (HCAs), another hard-to-pronounce carcinogen. It's your choice. I use both types for my grilling. To limit PAHs and HCAs, do this:

- **TRIM FAT FROM MEATS.** Less dripping means less smoke, which reduces PAHs.
- **MARINATE.** Soaking meat in balsamic vinegar and lemon juice reduces HCAs by 90 percent.
- **FLIP FREQUENTLY.** Studies have shown that turning meat frequently results in fewer HCAs.

SOME OTHER TIPS FOR BETTER GRILLING:

BEFORE GRILLING, allow your meat to come to near room temperature—not festering on a picnic table in the hot sun, but on a plate inside the house. Take it out of the fridge about 30 minutes before cooking to foster more even cooking. Cover it with plastic wrap so the houseflies won't crap on it.

TO GET THOSE COOL, PROFESSIONAL-LOOKING SEAR MARKS, cook one side of the meat halfway to its desired doneness and then rotate it 45 degrees and let it go the rest of the way. Repeat on the other side.

TREAT YOUR BARBECUE GUESTS to Mexican-style corn on the cob. Pull three-quarters of the husk off and discard, leaving a thin layer of husk. Pull back the remaining husk to remove the silk, but leave the husk attached. Pour about 1 teaspoon of olive oil into the palm of your hand and rub it into each ear of corn. Then sprinkle ½ teaspoon cumin, mixed with a pinch of salt, over the corn. Fold the attached husks back into place and grill the corn for 15 minutes on medium heat, turning occasionally. The corn is done when it's golden, with light brown grill marks, and smells wonderful.

WHEN IT'S SNOWING OUT, use a grill pan to get that great charcoal flavor and those cool crosshatch grill lines on meat. Or use a broiler, which is really just an inverted grill in disguise.

Perfect your pasta.

To make great pasta, avoid the three most common screwups, says Chef Mario Batali: "overcooking, oversaucing, and overthinking." His fool-proof plan:

1. **HEAT 2 TABLESPOONS EXTRA-VIRGIN OLIVE OIL** in a large skillet over medium-high heat. Add 2 garlic cloves, sliced thin, and toast lightly. Next add vegetables chopped into bite-size pieces (asparagus, artichokes, zucchini, parsnips, Swiss chard, mushrooms, cauliflower, broccoli). Cook for 10 minutes until caramelized. Season with salt and pepper.

2. **BRING A POT OF SALTED WATER TO A BOIL.** Add 8 ounces of dried spaghetti and cook for 1 minute less than the shortest time listed on the package.

3. **DRAIN THE PASTA,** reserving a cup of the cooking water. Toss the pasta in the pan with the vegetables and cook for 30 seconds. If the pasta is dry, add a bit of the cooking water. Toss in chopped fresh parsley, basil, and oregano and serve with grated Parmigiano-Reggiano cheese.

Stay sharp.

A $100 chef's knife slices tomatoes as quickly and effectively as this book does if it's dull. And it's a lot more dangerous. Buy a "diamond steel" and keep your knives razor sharp.

1. **PLANT THE STEEL UPRIGHT ON YOUR COUNTERTOP.** Hold your knife at a 20-degree angle to the steel. (To get the angle right, imagine putting a quarter between the blade and the steel.)

2. **START WITH THE HEEL OF THE BLADE** at the top of the steel. In a single motion, pull the knife down and back to your body, allowing the entire length of the blade to work across the steel.

3. **SHARPEN THE BACK OF THE KNIFE** (where you see the blade's emblem) six times and the front four times.

4. **TEST IT ON A TOMATO.** It should cut through cleanly on a single stroke.

5. **NEVER RUN IT THROUGH THE DISHWASHER.** Always hand-wash.

Get to know quinoa.

First learn how to pronounce this protein-and-fiber-rich grain: It's KEEN-wah. Then learn why and how to cook it. Quinoa is considered a "complete" protein, which means, like beef, eggs, and dairy, it contains all the essential amino acids your body needs to build muscle. With twice the protein of regular cereal grains, twice the fiber of brown rice, fewer carbohydrates, and even some healthy fats, it's one of the most nutritious foods on the planet. Cook it like pasta: Fill a large pot with water and bring to a boil. Add the quinoa, turn the heat to low, and cook until tender, about 20 minutes. Drain and serve—as you would rice. It works well in vegetable salads, as a risotto, even as an alternative to oatmeal (stir in some milk and spice it up with raisins, sugar, and cinnamon).

Make your own dressing.

Store-bought salad dressing is a waste of money. It's often a soup of unpronounceable preservatives and way too many calories. Make your own herb vinaigrette by whisking together 1 cup extra-virgin olive oil, 1 cup grated Parmesan cheese, 2 tablespoons white wine vinegar, ½ cup low-fat plain yogurt, 1 teaspoon dried herbs (such as basil, oregano, and thyme), 1 tablespoon Dijon mustard, plus salt and pepper to taste. Store in the fridge and whisk before each use.

Dry your meat and fish before cooking.

Take a paper towel and dab the extra surface moisture off your meat and fish. Otherwise, the moisture can create steam when it hits the heat, steaming the protein and impeding caramelization.

Try a crunchy condiment.

Skip the mayonnaise spread and moisten your turkey sandwich with ⅓ cup of coleslaw made with vinaigrette. It adds flavor, moisture, and texture, and the vinegar reduces the effect the sandwich bread will have on your blood sugar.

Mix the perfect cocktail sauce.

A good sauce for shrimp, clams, and other seafood should make your nose hairs stand at attention. Combine ½ cup ketchup; 1½ tablespoons prepared horseradish; 1 tablespoon lemon juice; 1½ teaspoons Worcestershire sauce; 1 clove garlic, minced; 2 tablespoons chopped dill, tarragon, or thyme; and 1 jalapeño pepper, chopped. Mix well.

CHAPTER 4

The New Abs Diet Breakfasts

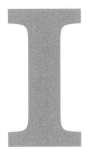

F YOU'RE LIKE MOST PEOPLE, here's what a typical workaday breakfast looks like.

6:30 A.M.: Stumble from bedroom into kitchen.

6:31 A.M.: Turn on light.

6:31:01 A.M.: Ouch! Curse light.

6:35 A.M.: Press button on coffee machine. Feel around in pantry for something that feels vaguely like a cereal box. Dump contents into bowl.

6:37 A.M.: Open fridge. Ouch! Curse light again. Grab milk.

6:38 A.M.: Pour milk into bowl.

6:40 A.M.: Spoon into mouth. Chew and swallow.

Ten minutes of boring repetition—the same coffee, the same cold cereal, the same milk stains on your bathrobe, week after week, month after month. It's no wonder so many of us just skip breakfast altogether. It's hard to get excited when you're eating the same meal in December that you were eating last January.

But while you may think that skipping breakfast is a way to cut calories, you're wrong. It's actually one of the best ways to add pounds to your frame. In fact, people who skip breakfast are 450 percent more likely to be obese than those who eat it on a regular basis, according to a study at the University of

Massachusetts Medical School. Why? Because eating breakfast wakes up your metabolism and starts your body burning calories. Think about it: You've been fasting for the past 8 to 10 hours since you ate last night's snack. While you were sleeping, your body's metabolism slowed down. By sacrificing breakfast when you wake up, you're operating on reserve fuel. Your body doesn't know there are eggs in the fridge; it thinks food is scarce so it throttles down your metabolism even further to protect you from starvation. As I mentioned in New Abs Diet Principal #2, skipping breakfast can actually cause your body to burn fewer calories all day long—by as much as 10 percent, according to nutritionist Leslie Bonci, M.P.H., RD, of the University of Pittsburgh Medical Center's Center for Sports Medicine, and a nutrition consultant to the Pittsburgh Steelers football team and Pittsburgh Pirates baseball team.

Plus, numerous studies show that those who eat breakfast actually consume fewer overall calories during the day. *The Journal of Nutrition* reports that eating protein for breakfast (think dairy, eggs, meat) leads to feelings of fullness that can last for hours. The morning meal may also reduce your risk of serious illnesses like heart disease, stroke, diabetes, and cancer, and it strengthens your immune system so you're more resistant to common ailments like colds and the flu, which are so easy to pick up at the workplace.

Okay, all good reasons to eat as soon as you wake. But it doesn't have to be the same cold cereal and milk every morning. Save that old standby for days when the alarm didn't go off or the kids have a cold or you need to shovel the driveway before you can get the car out. But on most other mornings, you'll have time to mix it up a bit. That's when you can utilize your kitchen to create the perfect start to your day. Try to get slow-burning carbohydrates, at least 20 grams of protein and 5 or more grams of fiber. That will provide your body with a high-quality, long-lasting, steady supply of energy to help you make it through the morning. Many of the meals on the following pages will deliver exactly what you need. But don't worry, they won't slow you down. I've included many speedy recipes that take minimal thinking, less than 3 minutes of prep, and won't require you to operate dangerous tools so early in the morning. Plus, I guarantee that these meals are way more nutritious (and tasty!) than those belly bombs they shovel at you through the drive-through window.

Quick Breakfast Tip

Within a half-hour of waking up, have a breakfast that includes high-quality protein and healthy fat to stabilize your blood sugar and help release endorphins to improve your mood. And don't forget about the slow-digesting carbohydrates like whole grain toast and oatmeal. Your carbohydrate resources are low after an overnight fast, so this is the best time to refuel your tank. Your brain needs a healthy dose of glucose from those carbohydrates to boost memory and concentration.

Turn the page for 34 New Abs Diet–approved recipes!

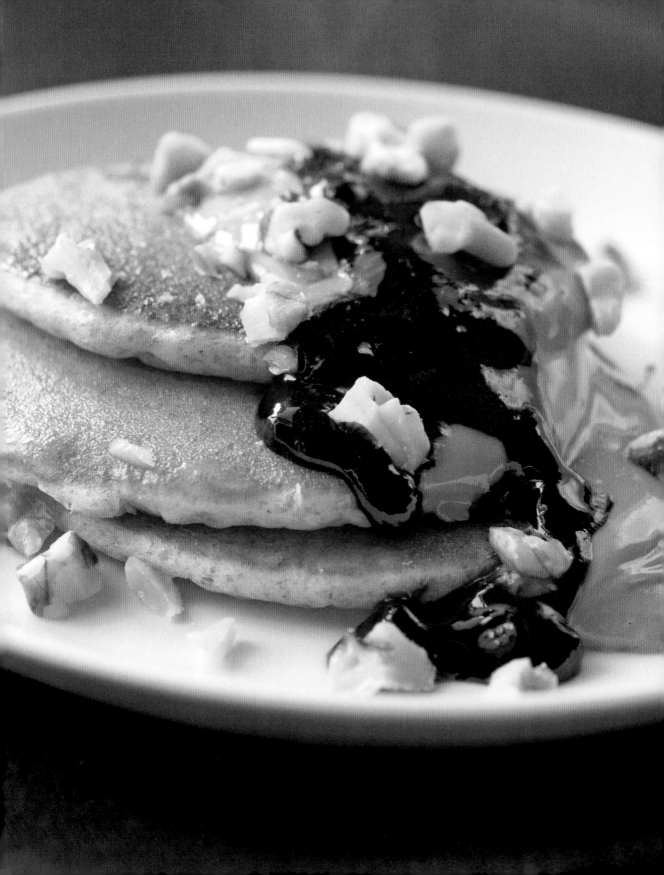

3-MINUTE MEAL **NO BATTER! NO BATTER!**
BLUEBERRY AND PEANUT BUTTER PANCAKE

Spike your brain with a morning hit of omega-3s by using omega-3-enriched peanut butter. Wash it down with a glass of fat-free milk. That adds 86 calories and 8 grams of protein. (Three servings shown.)
(Number of Powerfoods: 4)

1 FROZEN WHOLE WHEAT PANCAKE

2 TABLESPOONS OMEGA-3-ENRICHED PEANUT BUTTER

1 TABLESPOON BLUEBERRY PRESERVES OR A HANDFUL OF BLUEBERRIES

1 TABLESPOON CRUSHED WALNUTS

Heat the pancake in a toaster or toaster oven. Spread on the peanut butter, then top with the preserves and walnuts. Make it to go: Fold it in half like a taco and you won't even need a knife and fork.

Makes 1 serving.

Per serving: 360 calories, 12 g protein, 24 g carbohydrates, 26 g fat (3.5 g saturated), 300 mg sodium, 5 g fiber

WEEKEND BRUNCH

GOD-DIDN'T-MAKE-LITTLE-GREEN-APPLES HOME FRIES

Make these even better: Use skin-on diced new potatoes
for more nutrients and fiber. Serve with two fried eggs per serving.
(Number of Powerfoods: 2)

1½ TABLESPOONS BUTTER
 1 PACKAGE (24 OUNCES) DICED
   BREAKFAST POTATOES
½ POUND TURKEY STEAK, DICED
 1 LARGE GRANNY SMITH OR OTHER
   GREEN APPLE, CHOPPED
 1 TABLESPOON McCORMICK MONTREAL
   SEASONING OR CRACKED BLACK
   PEPPER AND PAPRIKA

Melt the butter in a large nonstick skillet over medium heat. Dump in the potatoes, turkey, and apple. Sprinkle with the seasoning mix. Stir to mix, then let cook for 5 minutes. Turn the mixture over with a spatula. Continue cooking for about 20 minutes, turning every few minutes to brown the potatoes on all sides.

Makes 6 servings.

Per serving: 360 calories, 12 g protein, 24 g carbohydrates, 26 g fat (3.5 g saturated), 300 mg sodium, 5 g fiber

2 fried eggs: add 180 calories, 13 g protein, 1 g carbohydrate, 14 g fat (4 g saturated), 190 mg sodium, 0 g fiber

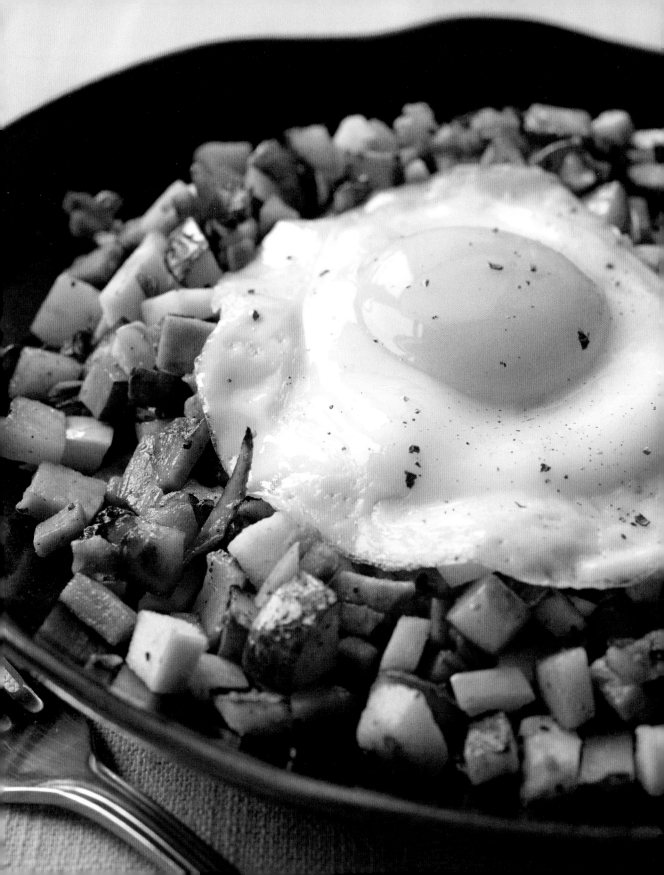

SPEEDY EATS

Grab these to-go breakfast snacks when you just have to catch that bus, train, carpool, or plane. Got kids? They'll enjoy them, too.

APPLE AND PEANUT POPS

- 1 MEDIUM APPLE
- 1 TUBE OF SQUEEZEABLE PEANUT BUTTER

Leave these on a chair by the door with your keys so you can grab them on your way out in the morning. Bite apple, squeeze some peanut butter into your mouth, chew, repeat. **280 calories**

BAM CRACKERS

- 1 TABLESPOON PEANUT BUTTER
- 1 LOW-FAT GRAHAM CRACKER, BROKEN IN HALF
- 4 DRIED PLUMS (PRUNES)

Spread peanut butter on both halves of the graham cracker. Arrange the prunes on 1 cracker half and top with the other. **190 calories**

BREAKFAST DOGS

- 1 TABLESPOON ALMOND BUTTER OR PEANUT BUTTER
- 1 WHOLE WHEAT HOT DOG ROLL
- 1 MEDIUM BANANA
- 1 TEASPOON HONEY
- 1 TABLESPOON GROUND FLAXSEED

Spread the nut butter on a split hot dog roll. Put the peeled banana in the roll, squeeze on some honey, and sprinkle with flaxseed. **390 calories**

COLD PIZZA WITH EXTRA PROTEIN

- 1 SLICE LEFTOVER COLD CHEESE PIZZA
- 2 SLICES LOX (SMOKED SALMON)

Admit it, you've eaten cold pizza for breakfast. Adding some lox makes it almost gourmet. **810 calories**

'COTTA GO

- 1 SLICE PUMPERNICKEL BREAD
- ½ CUP PART-SKIM RICOTTA CHEESE
- ½ CUP BLUEBERRIES, COARSELY CHOPPED GROUND CINNAMON

Toast the bread. Mix the ricotta and blueberries; spread on the toast. Sprinkle with cinnamon. **300 calories**

GUAC 'N' ROLL

- 1 MEDIUM WHOLE WHEAT TORTILLA
- 2 SLICES DELI TURKEY
- ¼ AVOCADO, PEELED AND SLICED

Top a tortilla with turkey and avocado and roll it up. **230 calories**

VEGGIE SAUSAGE WRAP

- 2 MORNINGSTAR FARMS VEGGIE SAUSAGES
- 1 MEDIUM WHOLE WHEAT TORTILLA
- ¼ CUP SHREDDED REDUCED-FAT MEXICAN-BLEND CHEESE

Nuke the veggie sausages for 45 seconds. Place them end-to-end in the tortilla and then top with the cheese, which will melt when you roll the tortilla. **300 calories**

YOGURT CONES

- ½ CUP GREEK YOGURT
- 1 HANDFUL MIXED NUTS AND SEEDS WAFER-STYLE ICE CREAM CONE

How to eat yogurt with your fingers: Mix the yogurt and nuts in a bowl and then spoon into the ice cream cone for a quick, calcium-and-protein-rich breakfast to go. **250 calories**

FIT FACT

Eat before you exercise. Putting something into your stomach before a morning workout prevents your muscle tissue from becoming cardio chow. Studies show that the body quickly starts burning muscle for energy once it has depleted its energy stores during exercise.

OVERTIME OATS

The steel-cut oats take some time to cook, but it's worth the wait; this is a breakfast that sticks with you.
(Number of Powerfoods: 3)

4½ CUPS WATER
 1 CUP STEEL-CUT OATS
½ CUP OAT BRAN
½ TEASPOON SALT
 18 WALNUT HALVES
 2 LARGE STRAWBERRIES, SLICED

Mix the water, oats, oat bran, and salt in a medium saucepan. Bring to a boil over medium-high heat. Reduce the heat and cover the pan. Simmer, stirring frequently, for 30 minutes or until thickened. Serve topped with the walnuts and strawberries.

Makes 3 1-cup servings.

Per serving: 220 calories, 8 g protein, 31 g carbohydrates, 11 g fat (1.5 g saturated), 400 mg sodium, 6 g fiber

ABS DIET HALL OF FAME
GREEN EGGS AND HAM OMELET
(Number of Powerfoods: 4)

 2 EGGS
 1 SLICE CANADIAN BACON, DICED
⅓ CUP TORN BABY SPINACH LEAVES
 1 TABLESPOON SHREDDED REDUCED-FAT SMOKED MOZZARELLA CHEESE

Whisk the eggs in a bowl, then stir in the Canadian bacon and spinach. Coat a nonstick skillet with cooking spray. Pour in the eggs, cook over medium heat until set, and flip. Sprinkle with the cheese and fold the omelet in half.

Makes 1 serving.

Per serving: 200 calories, 20 g protein, 3 g carbohydrates, 12 g fat (4.5 g saturated), 560 mg sodium, 0 g fiber

10-Second Blubber Buster
Your last-ditch opportunity for a morning jolt of binge-protection

If you don't have time to eat anything for breakfast, at least chug some milk. Doing so will likely help you eat less at lunch, say Australian scientists. In their study, overweight people who drank about 2½ cups of fat-free milk in the morning consumed 8.5 percent fewer calories at an all-you-can-eat lunch buffet than people who drank orange juice in the morning. What's the difference between the drinks? Milk has protein, which helps you feel fuller throughout the morning, while the OJ has no protein and lots of quick-burning sugar, which triggers hunger.

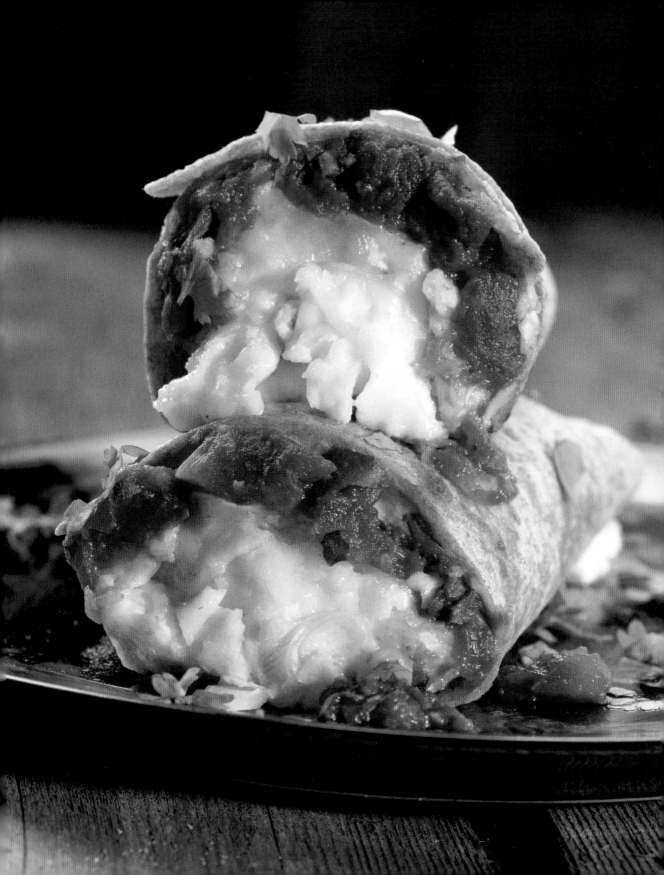

3-MINUTE MEAL **EL DESAYUNO WRAP**

Use a microwave to speed up this southwestern breakfast burrito.
(Number of Powerfoods: 3)

2 EGGS

1 SCALLION, SLICED

1 MEDIUM WHOLE WHEAT TORTILLA

2 TABLESPOONS SHREDDED REDUCED-
FAT MEXICAN-BLEND CHEESE

1 TABLESPOON CHOPPED CILANTRO

2 TABLESPOONS SALSA

HOT SAUCE (OPTIONAL)

Whisk the eggs and scallion in a microwavable bowl. Microwave for 2 minutes or until set. Spoon the eggs onto the tortilla; top with the shredded cheese, cilantro, salsa, and a squirt of hot sauce (if using). Roll up the tortilla and slice in half.

Makes 1 serving.

Per serving: 270 calories, 20 g protein, 24 g carbohydrates, 13 g fat (5 g saturated), 630 mg sodium, 3 g fiber

FRENCH TOAST, ITALIAN-STYLE

If you have time, let the ricotta come to room temp so it spreads easier.
(Number of Powerfoods: 4)

2 TABLESPOONS PART-SKIM RICOTTA CHEESE

2 SLICES WHOLE GRAIN BREAD

1 TEASPOON HONEY

1 TABLESPOON SLICED ALMONDS

½ TEASPOON GROUND CINNAMON

1 EGG

1 TABLESPOON 1 PERCENT MILK

HANDFUL OF FRESH BERRIES (STRAWBERRY, BLUEBERRY, BLACKBERRY)

1. Spread the ricotta on 1 bread slice. Drizzle the honey over the ricotta, top with the sliced almonds, and sprinkle lightly with cinnamon. Top with the remaining bread to form a sandwich.

2. Coat a nonstick griddle or skillet with cooking spray and heat over medium heat. Whisk the egg, milk, and any remaining cinnamon in a shallow bowl. Dip the sandwich into the egg to coat both sides. Place in the pan and cook until the bread is lightly browned on both sides. Serve with the berries.

Makes 1 serving.

Per serving: 330 calories, 18 g protein, 43 g carbohydrates, 10 g fat (3.5 g saturated), 340 mg sodium, 6 g fiber

FOOD FACT

Ricotta cheese is technically not a cheese at all because it's made from the whey (liquid) drained from other cheeses. But that makes it naturally low in fat and sodium, with a fat content of 4 to 10 percent. So put ricotta to good use other than in your Italian lasagna.

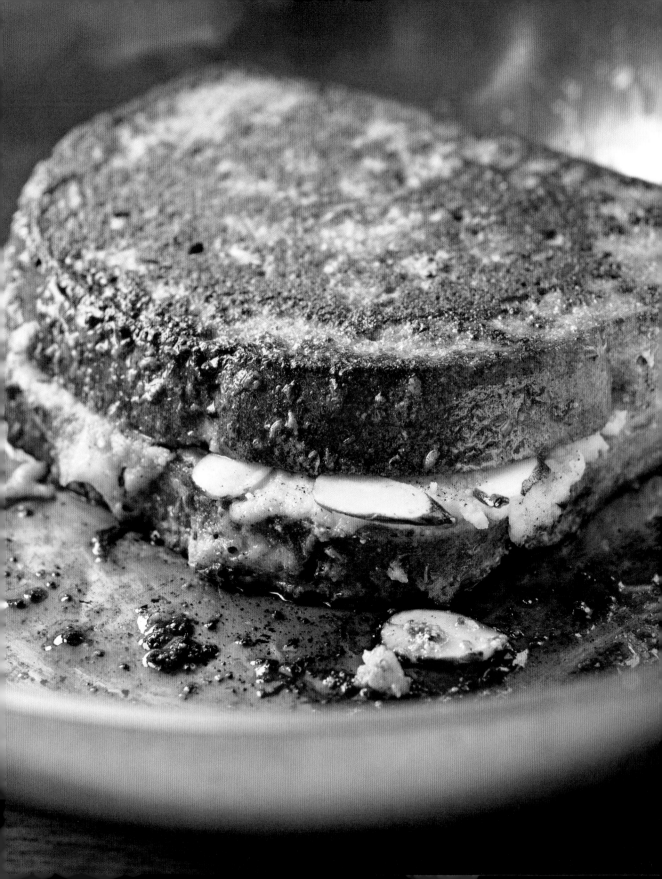

BLACK BEAN BREAKFAST QUESADILLAS
(Number of Powerfoods: 5)

1 CAN (24 OUNCES) BLACK BEANS, RINSED AND DRAINED

1 CUP SHREDDED REDUCED-FAT MONTEREY JACK CHEESE

1 JALAPEÑO OR SERRANO PEPPER, THINLY SLICED

8 SMALL WHOLE WHEAT TORTILLAS

2 TEASPOONS EXTRA-VIRGIN OLIVE OIL

1 AVOCADO, PITTED, PEELED, AND SLICED

½ LIME, CUT INTO WEDGES

1. Preheat the oven to 200°F. Divide the beans, cheese, and pepper evenly among 4 tortillas. Top with the remaining tortillas.

2. Heat 1 teaspoon oil in a large nonstick skillet over medium-high heat. Put 2 quesadillas in the pan. Press down with a spatula as they cook. Shake the pan so they don't stick. Brown for 2 to 4 minutes, flip, and cook the other side until browned and the cheese is melted. Move the finished quesadillas to the oven to keep warm. Then repeat the process with the remaining oil and quesadillas.

3. Cut the quesadillas into quarters with a pizza cutter or knife. Top each quarter with 2 avocado slices. Squeeze lime juice on top.

Makes 4 servings.

Per serving: 460 calories, 20 g protein, 56 g carbohydrates, 20 g fat (7 g saturated), 790 mg sodium, 15 g fiber

How to Open an Avocado

1. Using a sharp knife, slice the avocado lengthwise in half, starting with the thicker end and working the knife carefully around the pit (figure a). **2.** Hold the avocado in both hands, one on each side of the cut. Twist the halves in opposite directions to separate. **3.** With a forceful chop, whack the center of the knife blade into the pit, then twist and pull to remove (figure b). Toss the pit. **4.** Slice each avocado half lengthwise into two (figure c). **5.** Remove the peel and cut the avocado quarters into wedges or dice them (figure d).

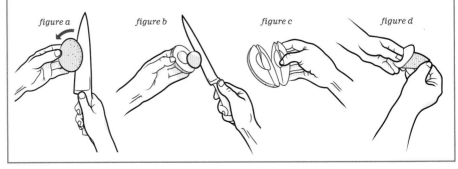

figure a   *figure b*   *figure c*   *figure d*

BREAKFAST PIZZA RUSTICA

Experiment with your own variations by using different vegetables, cheeses, and salsa.
(Number of Powerfoods: 5)

- 1 MINI WHOLE WHEAT PIZZA CRUST
- 1 HANDFUL OF MUSHROOMS, THINLY SLICED
- 1 HANDFUL OF BABY-SPINACH, ROUGHLY TORN
- 2 TABLESPOONS CRUMBLED GOAT CHEESE
- 2 TABLESPOONS OLIVE OIL
- 1 EGG
  SALT AND PEPPER TO TASTE

1. Preheat an oven to 350°F.

2. Top the pizza crust with the mushrooms, spinach, and goat cheese.

3. Drizzle the oil on top and crack an egg into the center of the pizza round.

4. Bake the pizza according to the package directions, or until the egg is cooked. To serve, quarter the pizza, allowing the yolk to break. Season with salt and pepper.

Makes 2 servings.

Per serving: 398 calories, 14.4 g protein, 33.9 g carbohydrates, 24 g fat (7 g saturated), 461 mg sodium, 6 g fiber

STOKE-YOUR-FIRE CEREAL

(Number of Powerfoods: 3)

- 1 CUP LOW-FAT VANILLA YOGURT
- 1 TEASPOON VANILLA WHEY PROTEIN POWDER
- ½ CUP ALL-BRAN CEREAL

Mix the yogurt and protein powder. Stir in the cereal.

Makes 1 serving.

Per serving: 300 calories, 19 g protein, 57 g carbohydrates, 4.5 g fat (2 g saturated), 240 mg sodium, 9 g fiber

ABS DIET HALL OF FAME
EGGS BENEFICIAL BREAKFAST SANDWICH

(Number of Powerfoods: 4)

- 1 EGG
- 3 EGG WHITES
- 1 TEASPOON GROUND FLAXSEED
- 2 SLICES WHOLE WHEAT BREAD, TOASTED
- 1 SLICE CANADIAN BACON
- 1 TOMATO, SLICED, OR 1 GREEN BELL PEPPER, SLICED

Mix the egg and egg whites in a bowl; add the flaxseed. Coat a skillet with cooking spray, scramble the eggs over medium heat, and dump onto the toast. Add the bacon and vegetable.

Makes 1 serving.

Per serving: 350 calories, 32 g protein, 33 g carbohydrates, 10 g fat (3 g saturated), 900 mg sodium, 7 g fiber

FOOD FACT
Canadian bacon, also called "back bacon," is leaner than pork-belly bacon because it comes from the loin of the pig. The appearance and flavor are closer to ham than the sizzling stuff. Two slices deliver just 89 calories and 11.7 grams of belly-satisfying protein.

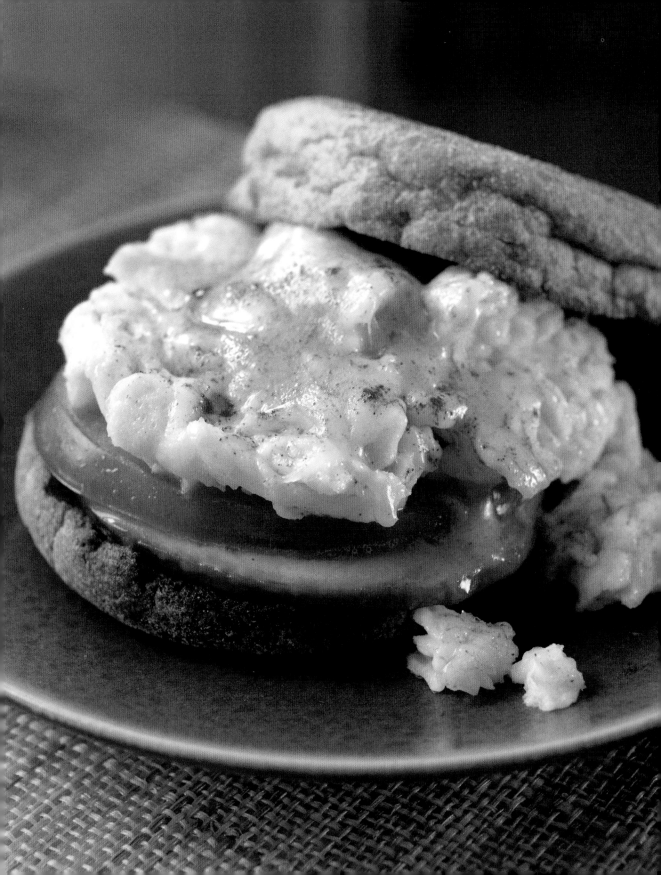

THE FOUR-COUNTRY BREAKFAST
(Number of Powerfoods: 4)

1 EGG, SCRAMBLED

1 SLICE CANADIAN BACON

1 WHOLE WHEAT ENGLISH MUFFIN,
SPLIT AND TOASTED

1 TABLESPOON SHREDDED REDUCED-FAT
MEXICAN-BLEND CHEESE

PINCH OF SWEET HUNGARIAN PAPRIKA

Arrange the egg and bacon on half of
the muffin. Top with the cheese and
paprika. Place the other muffin half on
top. Toast in a toaster oven until the
cheese melts.

Makes 1 serving.

Per serving: 270 calories, 20 g protein,
28 g carbohydrates, 10 g fat (3.5 g saturated) 800 mg sodium, 4 g fiber

ABS DIET HALL OF FAME
WHEY-TOO-EASY OATMEAL
(Number of Powerfoods: 4)

- 1 CUP 1 PERCENT MILK
- 1 CUP ROLLED OATS
- PINCH OF SALT
- PINCH OF GROUND CINNAMON
- 1 SCOOP VANILLA WHEY PROTEIN POWDER
- ½ CUP FRESH OR FROZEN BLUEBERRIES
- SPLENDA

Mix the milk, oats, salt, and cinnamon in a microwavable bowl. Microwave for 2 minutes, or until thick. Let cool slightly, then sprinkle evenly with the protein powder to avoid lumps and stir in. Stir in the blueberries and sweeten with Splenda.

Makes 1 serving.

Per serving: 570 calories, 38 g protein, 86 g carbohydrates, 10 g fat (3.5 g saturated), 310 g sodium, 10 g fiber

CAROLINA HOT GRITS
AND SAUSAGE
This 5-minute breakfast trims fat by using vegetarian "sausage."
(Number of Abs Diet Powerfoods: 2)

- 3 TABLESPOONS INSTANT GRITS
- 2 FULLY COOKED VEGETARIAN BREAKFAST SAUSAGE PATTIES, THAWED AND CRUMBLED
- ¾ CUP FAT-FREE MILK
- SALT AND GROUND BLACK PEPPER
- HOT SAUCE, TO TASTE
- 1 SLICE LOW-FAT CHEDDAR CHEESE

1. Combine the grits, sausage, and milk in a large microwavable bowl.

2. Cover with vented plastic wrap or a loose lid and microwave on high for 3 minutes, stirring halfway through cooking.

3. Season with salt, pepper, and hot sauce. Top with the cheese. Cover and microwave on high for 30 seconds or until the cheese has melted.

Makes 1 serving.

Per serving: 449 calories, 30 g protein, 40 g carbohydrate, 20 g fat (6.4 g saturated), 1,471 mg sodium, 3.6 g fiber

How to Pick a Better Yogurt
Some yogurts contain up to 36 grams of sugar per serving, about as much as a can of soda pop. Here are some tips for finding the best yogurt for your body.

SHOOT FOR MORE PROTEIN Greek yogurt contains up to 18 grams of protein per serving (three times the amount in some regular yogurts).

HUNT FOR CALCIUM Choose a yogurt that contains at least 20 percent of your daily calcium needs.

KEEP THE CALORIE COUNT AROUND 100 Plain yogurt contains a relatively small amount of natural sugar and hovers around 100 calories. The sweeter flavored fruit yogurts can contain 170 calories per serving.

MAKE IT BETTER If you want a sweeter yogurt, add a healthy sugar, like blueberries and raisins. Toss in some walnuts or almonds for added nutrition.

THE GREAT PUMPKIN BREAD
(Number of Powerfoods: 4)

1½ CUPS WHOLE WHEAT FLOUR
¾ CUP GROUND FLAXSEED
1 TEASPOON BAKING SODA
½ TEASPOON BAKING POWDER
½ TEASPOON SALT
½ TEASPOON GROUND NUTMEG
½ TEASPOON GROUND ALLSPICE
½ TEASPOON GROUND CINNAMON
¼ TEASPOON GROUND CLOVES
8 OUNCES CANNED
    UNSWEETENED PUMPKIN
½ CUP GRANULATED SUGAR
½ CUP PACKED BROWN SUGAR
½ CUP UNSWEETENED APPLESAUCE
1 EGG
1 EGG WHITE
⅓ CUP FAT-FREE MILK
½ CUP DRIED CRANBERRIES

1. Preheat the oven to 350°F.
Coat a 9-by-5-inch loaf pan with
cooking spray.

2. Mix the flour, flaxseed, baking soda,
baking powder, salt, and spices in a
large bowl. Whisk the pumpkin, sugars,
applesauce, eggs, and milk in a medium
bowl. Pour over the dry ingredients and
gently stir together. Fold in the
cranberries. Pour into the loaf pan.

3. Bake about 40 minutes, until a
toothpick inserted in the center comes
out clean. Let stand on a wire rack for
15 minutes. Turn out of the pan and
cool completely.

Makes 8 slices.

Per slice: 280 calories, 7 g protein,
57 g carbohydrates, 4.5 g fat
(0 g saturated), 360 mg sodium, 7 g fiber

ABS DIET HALL OF FAME
THE FLAX MACHINE
(Number of Powerfoods: 4)

1 CUP 1 PERCENT MILK
¾ CUP PLAIN INSTANT OATMEAL
½ BANANA, SLICED
1 TABLESPOON PEANUT BUTTER
1 TEASPOON HONEY
1 TEASPOON GROUND FLAXSEED
    PINCH OF BROWN SUGAR

Mix the milk and oatmeal in a
microwavable bowl. Microwave for
2 minutes or until thick. Stir in the
remaining ingredients.

Makes 1 serving.

Per serving: 400 calories, 18 g protein,
57 g carbohydrates, 13 g fat
(4 g saturated), 270 mg sodium, 6 g fiber

FOOD FACT
If you're trying to
cut calories from
baked goods, you
can substitute
applesauce for
some oils and other
fats. Like fats, the
pectin in the
applesauce keeps
the flour and water
from forming
gluten, which
results in a rubbery
final product.
As a general rule,
use half as much
applesauce as you
would oil. And
you'll get better
results if you don't
eliminate all the fat
in a baking recipe.

BACON AND EGG SALAD SANDWICH
Make the egg salad ahead. There's enough for four breakfast sandwiches,
lunches, or snacks.
(Number of Powerfoods: 4)

   6 EGGS
   ⅓ CUP SLICED CELERY
   ⅓ CUP LIGHT MAYONNAISE
      SALT AND PEPPER
   2 SLICES WHOLE GRAIN BREAD
   2 SLICES COOKED TURKEY BACON
   2 GREEN LEAF LETTUCE LEAVES
   1 SLICE TOMATO

1. Place the whole eggs in a large saucepan and cover with 1½ quarts of water. Bring to a simmer over high heat. Immediately shut off the burner and wait 10 minutes. Drain and run cold water over the eggs to stop cooking.

2. Peel the eggs and chop. Combine with the celery and mayonnaise; season with salt and pepper. Refrigerate overnight.

3. In the morning: Toast the bread while heating the bacon in a microwave. Spread 2 tablespoons egg salad on 1 toast slice and top with the bacon, lettuce, tomato, and remaining toast. Refrigerate remaining egg salad for other meals.

Makes 1 serving.

Per serving: 220 calories, 12 g protein, 9 g carbohydrates, 14 g fat (3.5 g saturated), 440 mg sodium, 1 g fiber

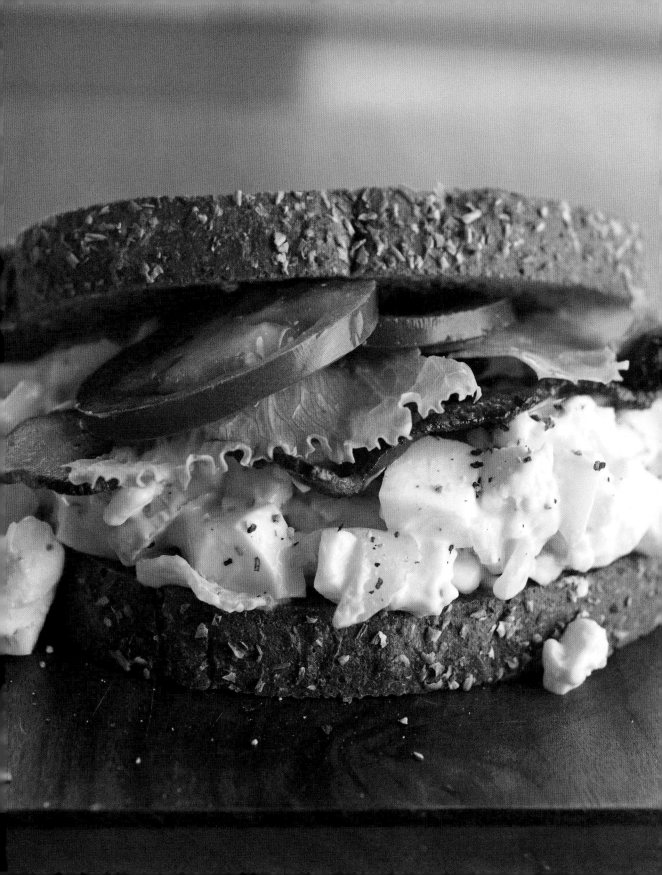

DINNER-FOR-BREAKFAST BURRITO

Here's a super use for leftover chicken. Eat it with a cup of cottage cheese topped with a handful of blueberries.
(Number of Powerfoods: 6)

1 MEDIUM WHOLE WHEAT TORTILLA

1 COOKED CHICKEN BREAST, SLICED

¼ CUP SHREDDED REDUCED-FAT MONTEREY JACK CHEESE

¼ CUP JARRED SOUTHWESTERN BLACK BEAN AND CORN SALSA

Warm the tortilla in a nonstick skillet. Microwave the chicken on a plate for 30 seconds to warm it and place on the tortilla. Top with the cheese and salsa. Roll up.

Makes 1 serving.

Per serving (with cottage cheese and blueberries): 530 calories, 48 g protein, 48 g carbohydrates, 16.5 g fat (6.5 g saturated), 1,460 mg sodium, 8 g fiber

ABS DIET HALL OF FAME
HONEY, I SHRUNK MY GUT

(Number of Powerfoods: 5)

1 CUP 1 PERCENT MILK

¾ CUP PLAIN INSTANT OATMEAL

½ CUP BLUEBERRIES OR BLACKBERRIES

1 TABLESPOON CHOPPED WALNUTS OR PECANS

1 TEASPOON HONEY

1 TEASPOON GROUND FLAXSEED

PINCH OF GROUND CINNAMON

Mix the milk and oatmeal in a microwavable bowl. Microwave for 2 minutes or until thick. Stir in the remaining ingredients.

Makes 1 serving.

Per serving: 340 calories, 15 g protein, 52 g carbohydrates, 10 g fat (2.5 g saturated), 190 mg sodium, 6 g fiber

FOOD FACT

Precooked chicken breasts will make your life easier if you always have them on hand. Shred them and toss into salads. Chop and add to pasta dishes. Nuke a cooked breast and add to instant brown rice and steamed broccoli for a meal in less than 5 minutes. Whenever you grill, bake, or broil chicken, make extra. Let cool, wrap in plastic, and toss into the refrigerator. They will be there ready for you when you don't have the time or the desire to cook.

FLAPJACKS WITH CHOCOLATE CHIPS
(Number of Powerfoods: 4)

¾ CUP WHOLE WHEAT FLOUR
1 TABLESPOON BAKING POWDER
1 TEASPOON SALT
1½ CUPS 2 PERCENT MILK
1 CUP PLAIN INSTANT OATMEAL
1 TABLESPOON BROWN SUGAR
1 TEASPOON VANILLA EXTRACT
2 EGGS, LIGHTLY BEATEN
½ CUP CHOCOLATE CHIPS

1. Mix the flour, baking powder, and salt in a small bowl. Mix the milk, oatmeal, sugar, and vanilla in a large bowl. Stir in the eggs and then add the dry ingredients, a little at a time. Stir in the chocolate chips.

2. Coat a griddle or nonstick skillet with cooking spray and heat over medium-high heat. Using a measuring cup, pour about ¼ cup of batter onto the hot surface for each pancake. When the edges of the pancakes are cooked and little bubbles form in the middle, flip the pancakes over. Cook until golden brown.

Makes about 10 pancakes.

Per pancake: 140 calories, 5 g protein, 20 carbohydrates, 5 g fat (2.5 g saturated), 430 mg sodium, 2 g fiber

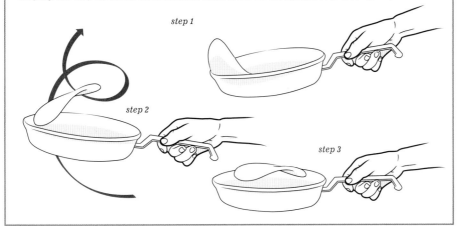

How to Flip a Flapjack

To turn a pancake over in the air with a flourish, sweep the skillet forward, up, and around in a smooth looping-the-loop motion. (Practice once or twice alone before trying to impress anyone.)

step 1

step 2

step 3

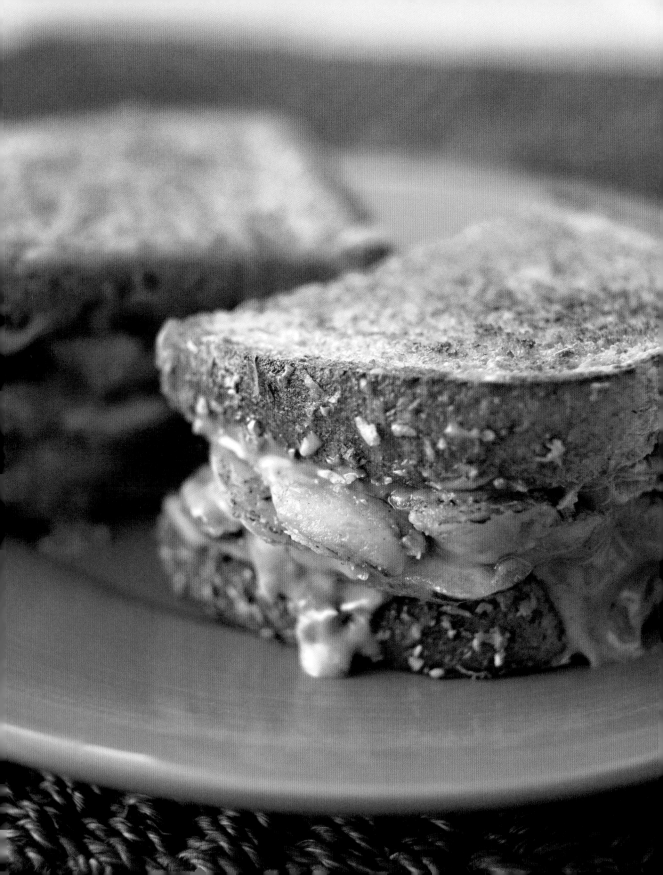

GRILLED BANANA SANDWICHES

Got kids? Want them to eat breakfast? Make this.
(Number of Powerfoods: 3)

1 LARGE BANANA

1½ TABLESPOONS LOW-FAT WHIPPED
CREAM CHEESE

1½ TABLESPOONS PEANUT BUTTER

1 TABLESPOON HONEY
PINCH OF SALT

4 SLICES WHOLE GRAIN BREAD

1. Cut off one-quarter of the banana and mash in a bowl with a fork; stir in the cream cheese, peanut butter, honey, and salt. Spread over 2 bread slices.

2. Coat a large skillet with cooking spray and place over medium-high heat. Slice the remaining banana in half lengthwise and then in half crosswise. Place the banana halves in the pan and cook until caramelized. Arrange the bananas over the cream cheese and top with the remaining bread.

3. Wipe out the skillet, add a spritz more cooking spray, and place over medium heat. Add the sandwiches and cook until browned on each side.

Makes 2 servings.

Per serving: 320 calories, 11 g protein, 50 g carbohydrates, 10 g fat (2 g saturated), 320 mg sodium, 6 g fiber

ABS DIET HALL OF FAME **THE ULTIMATE POWER BREAKFAST**

More power hitters than the Yankees' batting lineup.
And still you can knock this out of the park in less than 5 minutes!
(Number of Powerfoods: 8)

1 EGG

1 CUP 1 PERCENT MILK

¾ CUP PLAIN INSTANT OATMEAL

½ CUP MIXED BERRIES

1 TABLESPOON CHOPPED PECANS
   OR SLICED ALMONDS

1 TEASPOON VANILLA WHEY
   PROTEIN POWDER

1 TEASPOON GROUND FLAXSEED

½ BANANA, SLICED

1 TABLESPOON PLAIN YOGURT

Whisk everything but the banana and yogurt in a microwavable bowl. Microwave for 2 minutes or until set. Let cool for a minute or two. Top with the banana and yogurt.

Makes 1 serving.

Per serving: 570 calories, 29 g protein, 80 g carbohydrates, 18 g fat (4.5 g saturated), 200 mg sodium, 11 g fiber

FOOD FACT

The calcium in milk may increase the rate at which your body burns fat, according to a study at the University of Tennessee.

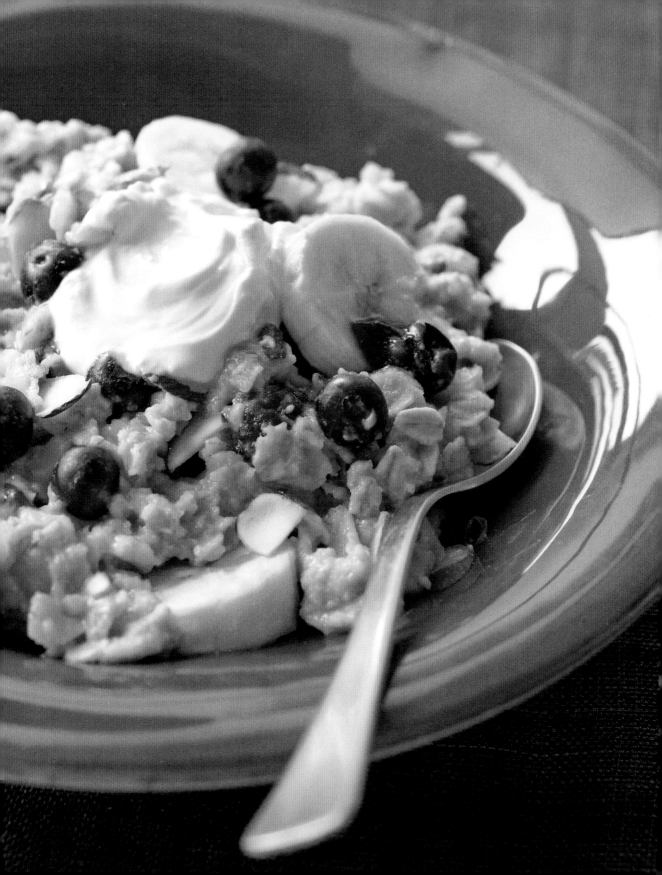

A GUAC IN THE PARK BREAKFAST BURRITO
(Number of Powerfoods: 5)

2 EGGS
FAT-FREE MILK
PINCH OF BLACK PEPPER
2 SLICES FAT-FREE TURKEY DELI SLICES
1 MEDIUM WHOLE WHEAT TORTILLA
2 TABLESPOONS SHREDDED REDUCED-FAT MEXICAN-BLEND CHEESE
½ AVOCADO, PEELED AND SLICED
SALSA (OPTIONAL)

Whisk the eggs, a shot of milk, and pepper in a microwavable bowl. Microwave for 2 minutes or until set. Place the turkey on the tortilla, add the eggs, and then top with the cheese, avocado, and salsa (if using). Roll up.

Makes 1 serving.

Per serving: 440 calories, 25 g protein, 30 g carbohydrates, 29 g fat (7 g saturated), 640 mg sodium, 9 g fiber

SALMON AND EGGS BREAKFAST BURRITO
(Number of Powerfoods: 5)

2 EGGS
1 SCALLION, SLICED
1 CUP CHOPPED BABY SPINACH LEAVES
1 TABLESPOON LOW-FAT CREAM CHEESE
1 MEDIUM WHOLE WHEAT TORTILLA
1 OUNCE SMOKED SALMON, TORN INTO PIECES

Whisk the eggs and stir in the scallion and spinach. Coat a nonstick skillet with cooking spray, add the eggs, and lightly scramble over medium heat. Spread the cream cheese on the tortilla. Top with the eggs and salmon. Fold the outer edges in, then roll.

Makes 1 serving.

Per serving: 360 calories, 35 g protein, 27 g carbohydrates, 15 g fat (5 g saturated), 400 mg sodium, 4 g fiber

Burn Calories in the Kitchen

Exercise while making breakfast. Crank out a few sets of three-way lunges and jump-start your metabolism. It's a great way to exercise the big calorie-burning muscles in your legs while improving mobility and stability in your hips. Here's how:

1. Step forward with your right leg, bending your right knee at a 90-degree angle. Simultaneously lower your hips toward the floor by bringing your left knee close to the ground.

2. Return to the starting position and then immediately step to your right into a wide base. Bend your right knee while keeping your left leg straight, shifting your hips to the right and down.

3. Return to the starting position and step backward with your right leg, lowering your hips toward the floor and bringing your right knee close to the ground while bending your left knee to nearly 90 degrees.

4. Repeat this series of lunges six times, holding each lunge for 2 seconds. Then repeat the exercise using your left leg to lunge. By the time you finish, your oats will be ready to eat.

A BANANA SPLIT BREAKFAST
(Number of Powerfoods: 3)

½ TEASPOON SUGAR

2 TABLESPOONS WATER

1 CUP FROZEN BLUEBERRIES

1 MEDIUM BANANA

4 OUNCES LOW-FAT VANILLA-FLAVORED GREEK YOGURT

¼ CUP CHOPPED WALNUTS

1. Stir the sugar, water, and frozen berries in a saucepan over medium-high heat. Bring to a boil, then reduce heat and simmer for 5 minutes.

2. Slice the banana in half lengthwise and place in a bowl. Spoon the vanilla yogurt over the banana halves. Pour the blueberry mixture over the bananas and yogurt and top with the walnuts.

Makes 1 serving.

Per serving: 470 calories, 13 g protein, 66 g carbohydrates, 21 g fat (3 g saturated), 85 mg sodium, 9 g fiber

ABS DIET HALL OF FAME
THE I-HAVEN'T-HAD-MY-COFFEE-YET SANDWICH
(Number of Powerfoods: 3)

1½ TEASPOONS LOW-FAT CREAM CHEESE

1 WHOLE WHEAT PITA, HALVED TO MAKE 2 POCKETS

2 SLICES TURKEY OR HAM

LETTUCE OR GREEN VEGETABLE

Spread cream cheese in the pockets of the pita. Stuff with meat and vegetables.

Makes 1 serving.

Per serving: 225 calories, 10 g protein, 42 g carbohydrates, 3 g fat (1 g saturated), 430 mg sodium, 6 g fiber

THE INCREDIBLE VEGETABLE OMELET
(Number of Powerfoods: 5)

2 TEASPOONS OLIVE OIL

½ CUP CHOPPED FROZEN SPINACH

½ CUP SLICED MUSHROOMS

½ CUP CHOPPED RED OR YELLOW BELL PEPPER

2 TABLESPOONS CHOPPED ONION

3 EGG WHITES, BEATEN

¼ CUP LOW-FAT SHREDDED CHEESE

1 SLICE WHOLE GRAIN TOAST

1 TEASPOON CANOLA OIL MARGARINE

1. Heat the olive oil in a fry pan over medium heat. Add all the vegetables and cook for 5 minutes until the mushrooms and peppers are tender and the onion is translucent. Move the vegetables to a plate.

2. Add the egg whites to the fry pan. Cook about 3 minutes until set. Top half of the egg with the vegetables from the plate. Fold the omelet over and cook for another minute or two.

3. Plate the omelet and top with the shredded cheese. Serve with wheat toast spread with canola margarine.

Makes 1 serving.

Per serving: 325 calories, 22 g protein, 20 g carbohydrates, 20 g fat (4 g saturated), 523 mg sodium, 6 g fiber

CHAPTER 5

The New Abs Diet Smoothies and Snacks

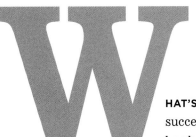

HAT'S MADE THE ABS DIET so successful for so many years has been its one simple, but revolutionary, idea: If you want to weigh less, you need to eat more.

Sure, it sounds crazy—the math doesn't seem to work when you shorthand it in your head. But consider this: The number-one predictor of whether you'll gain weight over the next 5 years is whether or not you're on a diet right now. The more you diet, the fatter you get. Period.

The wild card in this quest for weight loss is our hormonal system. When we diet and then binge, our insulin levels go crazy; insulin is the hormone responsible for managing blood sugar and telling us when we're weak with hunger. Leptin, the hormone that tells us when we're full, can be undermined by too much or too little food at any given time, especially some sugars. And cortisol, the fight-or-flight hormone, causes us to store fat when we're under stress (and what's more stressful than starving yourself?). It's not about cutting calories; cutting calories too severely leads to weight gain. Instead, it's about managing calories.

That's why, if you're following the New Abs Diet, you'll never go hungry. Because hunger is your enemy—it causes you to binge on food, it causes you to store more of the food you do eat as fat, and it decreases the number of calories you're burning during the day, another factor in weight gain.

And how do you keep hunger at bay? By snacking throughout the day. As I mentioned earlier, a study in the *American Journal of Epidemiology* found that people who ate four to six small meals a day were half as likely to become overweight as people who ate three or fewer times. And hence, this chapter.

Of course, when I say "snacks," I don't mean potato chips and onion dip. Good snacks are those that contain protein and a little bit of fat, like turkey, cheese, peanut butter, and nuts. Both nutrients are satiating, and they take longer to burn off, which keeps your blood sugar levels from taking roller-coaster rides. Other good snacks are fiber-rich foods like whole grains and foods that contain a high volume of water, like vegetables and fruit. And then there's my personal favorite: smoothies.

Smoothies are one of the staples of the Abs Diet for several reasons:

- Nutrition: A typical yogurt-based smoothie with some fruit gives you a wallop of protein and fiber and a ton of vitamins and minerals.
- Weight loss: A study at the University of Tennessee found that men who added three servings of yogurt a day to their diets lost 61 percent more body fat and 81 percent more stomach fat over 12 weeks than those who didn't eat yogurt. Another study showed that probiotic yogurt with live active cultures can change how much fat is available for the body to absorb by influencing stomach acids during digestion.
- Taste: You want a dessert that's healthy but tastes like berries and cream? How about one that tastes like peanut butter and chocolate? How about a daiquiri? You can do it all with the smoothie recipes in this chapter.
- Laziness: Really. If Jimmy Buffett can master a blender, so can you. It's as simple as tossing stuff in a bucket and pressing a button!

Try working the smoothies and snacks on the following pages into your day and watch the weight melt off.

Quick Snacks Tip

Those snack foods in 100-calorie packages may not help you lose weight. That's because if you're not full after finishing the package, you are likely to open another package, say researchers who study satiety. You will be better off, nutritionists say, if you consume snacks that are high in protein and fiber, like cheese, lean meat, and whole grain bread, and foods with high water volume, like fruits and vegetables, which keep you full with fewer calories.

Turn the page for 41 New Abs Diet–approved recipes!

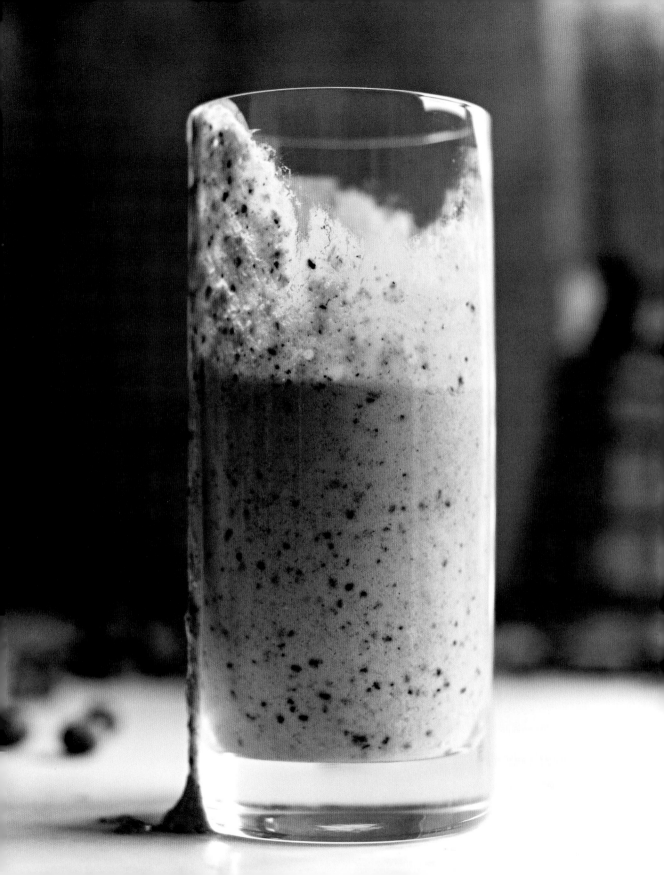

ABS DIET HALL OF FAME
HALLE BERRIES SMOOTHIE
(Number of Powerfoods: 4)

¾ CUP INSTANT OATMEAL NUKED
IN WATER OR FAT-FREE MILK

¾ CUP FAT-FREE MILK

¾ CUP FROZEN BLUEBERRIES,
STRAWBERRIES, AND RASPBERRIES

2 TEASPOONS VANILLA WHEY
PROTEIN POWDER

3 ICE CUBES

Dump the cooked oatmeal, milk, berries, whey powder, and ice into a blender, and puree until drinkable. (For a sweeter smoothie, add honey to taste.)

Makes 2 servings.

Per serving: 144 calories, 7 g protein, 27 g carbohydrates, 1 g fat (0 g saturated), 109 mg sodium, 4 g fiber

BLUE CHEESECAKE
(Number of Powerfoods: 6)

1 SCOOP LOW-FAT VANILLA ICE CREAM
½ CUP PART-SKIM RICOTTA CHEESE
½ CUP 1 PERCENT MILK
1 TABLESPOON VANILLA WHEY
  PROTEIN POWDER
2 TABLESPOONS LOW-FAT PLAIN YOGURT
½ CUP FROZEN BLUEBERRIES
3 ICE CUBES

Makes 1 serving.

Per serving: 400 calories, 28 g protein,
44 g carbohydrates, 14 g fat
(8 g saturated), 307 mg sodium, 3 g fiber

ARTERY AID
(Number of Powerfoods: 2)

8 OUNCES LOW-FAT VANILLA YOGURT
2 TABLESPOONS GROUND FLAXSEED
1 CUP SLICED FRESH OR FROZEN
  PEACHES
  HONEY TO TASTE

Makes 1 serving.

Per serving: 407 calories, 17 g protein,
65 g carbohydrates, 11 g fat
(0 g saturated), 100 mg sodium, 7 g fiber

Quick Pick Snack Mix

Healthy snacking doesn't require measuring spoons. For no-brainer snack prep, just grab something from column A (carbohydrates) and pair it with an item in column B (protein/fat).

COLUMN A	COLUMN B
Baby carrots	1 cup low-fat yogurt
4 dates	1-inch square Cheddar cheese
1 pear	1 stick low-fat string cheese
4 whole wheat crackers	1 tablespoon hummus
Celery sticks	1 tablespoon natural peanut butter
Whole wheat tortilla	2 slices turkey breast
Whole wheat breadstick	1 cup low-fat chocolate milk
½ cup blueberries	1 cup Greek yogurt
1 cup diced bell pepper	½ cup low-fat cottage cheese
1 slice whole grain bread	1 tablespoon almond butter
6 ounces orange juice	1 hard-cooked egg
4 strawberries	10 almonds
Broccoli florets	2 tablespoons low-fat ranch dressing

THE ORANGEMAN
(Number of Powerfoods: 3)

- 1 CUP 1 PERCENT MILK
- ½ CUP FROZEN ORANGE JUICE CONCENTRATE
- 2 TABLESPOONS LOW-FAT PLAIN YOGURT
- 1 BANANA
- 2 TEASPOONS WHEY PROTEIN POWDER
- 6 ICE CUBES

Makes 2 servings.

Per serving: 241 calories, 10 g protein, 48 g carbohydrates, 2 g fat (1 g saturated), 84 mg sodium, 2 g fiber

WHEY-GG NOG

- 1 CUP 1 PERCENT MILK
- 1 SCOOP VANILLA WHEY PROTEIN POWDER
- 1 GRAHAM CRACKER, BROKEN
- ½ TEASPOON GROUND ALLSPICE
- 4 ICE CUBES

Makes 1 serving.

Per serving: 170 calories, 18 g protein, 17 g carbohydrates, 3 g fat (1 g saturated), 130 mg sodium, 1 g fiber

ALMOND JOY
(Number of Powerfoods: 4)

- 6 OUNCES ORGANIC FAT-FREE MILK
- 1 TABLESPOON ALMOND BUTTER
- 1 SCOOP CHOCOLATE WHEY PROTEIN POWDER
- ½ BANANA
- 1 TEASPOON GROUND FLAXSEED
- 5 ICE CUBES

Makes 1 serving.

Per serving: 330 calories, 29 g protein, 30 g carbohydrates, 12 g fat (1.5 g saturated), 210 mg sodium, 3 g fiber

LIQUID SANDWICH
(Number of Powerfoods: 4)

- 1 CUP FAT-FREE MILK
- 1 BANANA
- ½ CUP RASPBERRIES
- ½ CUP FAT-FREE FROZEN YOGURT
- 1 TABLESPOON PEANUT BUTTER

Makes 1 serving.

Per serving: 410 calories, 19 g protein, 69 g carbohydrates, 9 g fat (1 g saturated), 242 mg sodium, 8 g fiber

COCO POOF
(Number of Powerfoods: 4)

- 1 SCOOP LOW-FAT CHOCOLATE ICE CREAM
- ½ CUP FROZEN RASPBERRIES
- ½ CUP 1 PERCENT CHOCOLATE MILK
- 1 TABLESPOON CHOCOLATE WHEY PROTEIN POWDER
- ½ BANANA
- 3 ICE CUBES

Makes 1 serving.

Per serving: 340 calories, 17 g protein, 56 g carbohydrates, 7 g fat (4 g saturated), 145 mg sodium, 6 g fiber

BEACHSIDE BLEND
(Number of Powerfoods: 1)

- 1 CUP PINEAPPLE ORANGE JUICE
- ½ CUP FRESH OR FROZEN MANGO CHUNKS
- ½ CUP FROZEN BLUEBERRIES
- 3 ICE CUBES

Makes 1 serving.

Per serving: 220 calories, 4 g protein, 54 g carbohydrates, 1 g fat (0 g saturated), 11 mg sodium, 3 g fiber

FIT FACT

It's hard to eat a cannoli when you're snoring. That may be why people who sleep a full 7 to 8 hours tend to be leaner. Researchers at University of Chicago found that people who lost 3 hours of slumber ate about 200 more calories (from snacks) the next day than they did when they got adequate sleep.

VIRGIN CABO DAIQUIRI
(Number of Powerfoods: 3)

½ CUP 1 PERCENT MILK

2 TABLESPOONS LOW-FAT PLAIN YOGURT

¼ CUP FROZEN ORANGE JUICE
   CONCENTRATE

½ BANANA

¼ CUP STRAWBERRIES

½ CUP CUBED MANGO

2 TEASPOONS VANILLA WHEY
   PROTEIN POWDER

3 ICE CUBES

Makes 2 servings.

Per serving: 154 calories, 7 g protein, 31 g carbohydrates, 1 g fat (0.5 g saturated), 50 mg sodium, 2 g fiber

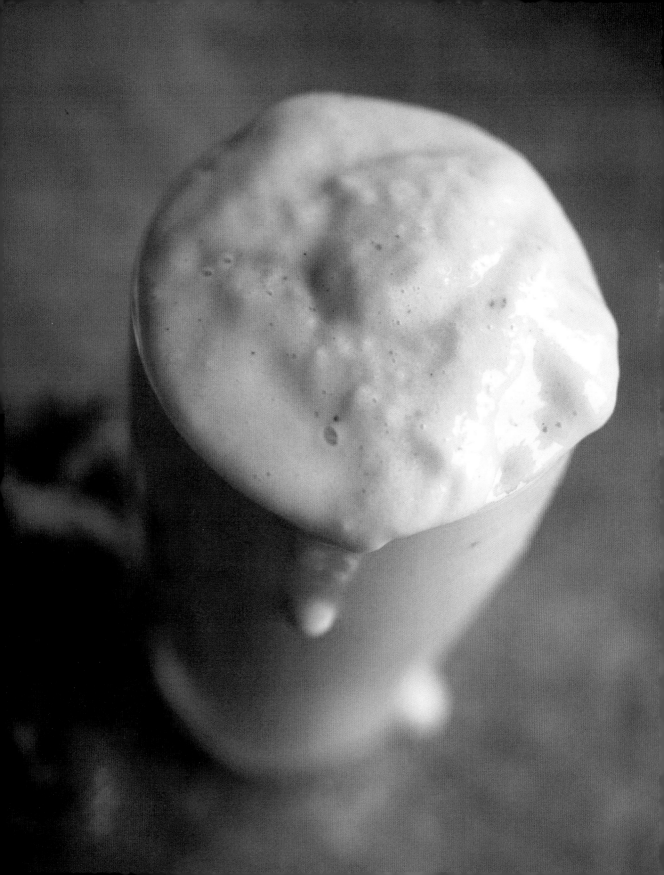

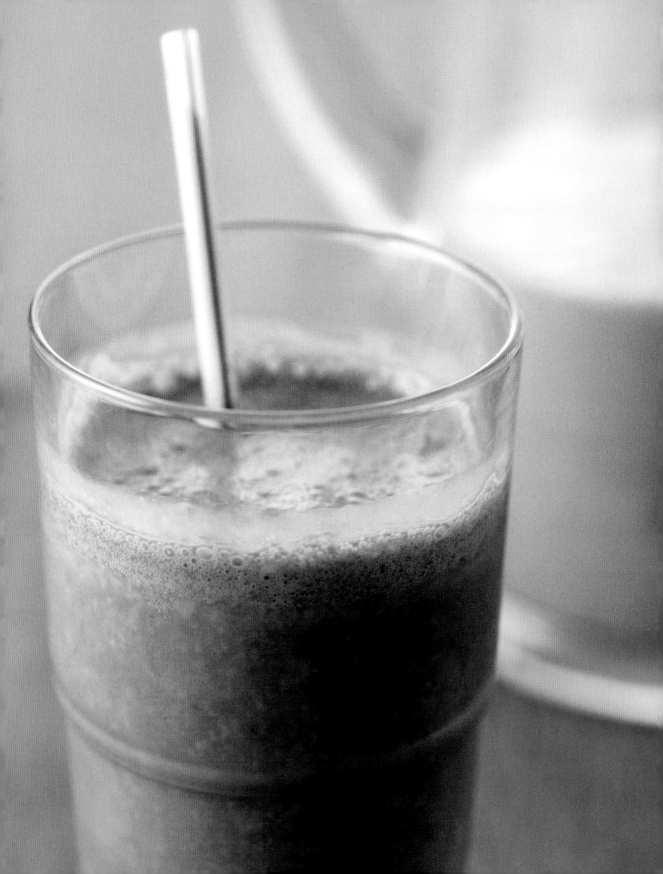

EXTREME CHOCOLATE
(Number of Powerfoods: 3)

- 1 SCOOP LOW-FAT CHOCOLATE ICE CREAM
- 1 TABLESPOON CHOCOLATE SYRUP
- ½ CUP 1 PERCENT CHOCOLATE MILK
- 1 TABLESPOON CHOCOLATE WHEY PROTEIN POWDER
- ½ BANANA
- 3 ICE CUBES

Makes 1 serving.

Per serving: 355 calories, 17 g protein, 60 g carbohydrates, 6 g fat (4 g saturated), 158 mg sodium, 4 g fiber

A LITTLE PEANUT BRITTLE SHAKE
(Number of Powerfoods: 3)

2 SCOOPS VANILLA WHEY PROTEIN POWDER

1 TABLESPOON INSTANT SUGAR-FREE BUTTERSCOTCH PUDDING MIX

¾ CUP FAT-FREE MILK

6 ICE CUBES

1 TABLESPOON CHUNKY PEANUT BUTTER

Put everything but the peanut butter in the blender and mix until smooth. Add the peanut butter and blend for just a few seconds to retain some chunkiness.

Makes 1 serving.

Per serving: 460 calories, 43 g protein, 44 g carbohydrates, 11 g fat (3 g saturated), 530 mg sodium, 1 g fiber

PEACHES EN REGALIA
(Number of Powerfoods: 4)

1 CUP 1 PERCENT MILK

2 TABLESPOONS LOW-FAT VANILLA YOGURT

½ CUP FROZEN PEACHES

½ CUP STRAWBERRIES

2 TEASPOONS VANILLA WHEY PROTEIN POWDER

3 ICE CUBES

Makes 2 servings.

Per serving: 152 calories, 9 g protein, 27 g carbohydrates, 2 g fat (1 g saturated), 83 mg sodium, 2 g fiber

TIRAMI-SMOOTH
(Number of Powerfoods: 5)

¾ CUP PART-SKIM RICOTTA CHEESE

2 TABLESPOONS LOW-FAT PLAIN YOGURT

1 TABLESPOON SLIVERED ALMONDS

2 TEASPOONS CHOCOLATE WHEY PROTEIN POWDER

2 TEASPOONS GROUND FLAXSEED

½ TEASPOON FINELY GROUND INSTANT COFFEE POWDER

6 ICE CUBES

Makes 2 servings.

Per serving: 207 calories, 15 g protein, 15 g carbohydrates, 10 g fat (5 g saturated), 134 mg sodium, 2 g fiber

OKAY ON THE OJ
(Number of Powerfoods: 4)

1 SCOOP LOW-FAT ORANGE SHERBET

½ CUP CANTALOUPE CHUNKS

½ CUP PART-SKIM RICOTTA CHEESE

½ CUP 1 PERCENT MILK

½ CUP ORANGE JUICE

1 TABLESPOON VANILLA WHEY PROTEIN POWDER

3 ICE CUBES

Makes 1 serving.

Per serving: 438 calories, 25 g protein, 60 g carbohydrates, 12 g fat (8 g saturated), 290 mg sodium, 1 g fiber

FIT FACT
Curb your hunger with a cardio appetizer. Research shows that running and strength training boost the body's production of the peptide YY (an appetite depressant) and curtail the production of ghrelin (an appetite stimulant).

STRAWBERRY SHORTCUT

(Number of Powerfoods: 4)

- 1 SCOOP LOW-FAT STRAWBERRY ICE CREAM
- ½ CUP FROZEN STRAWBERRIES
- ½ BANANA
- ½ CUP 1 PERCENT MILK
- 1 TABLESPOON VANILLA WHEY PROTEIN POWDER
- 3 ICE CUBES

Makes 1 serving.

Per serving: 283 calories, 14 g protein, 48 g carbohydrates, 4 g fat (2 g saturated), 106 mg sodium, 5 g fiber

PUMPKIN YOU UP!

(Number of Powerfoods: 3)

- 1 SCOOP LOW-FAT BUTTER PECAN ICE CREAM
- ½ CUP UNSWEETENED CANNED PUMPKIN
- ½ CUP 1 PERCENT MILK
- 1 TABLESPOON VANILLA WHEY PROTEIN POWDER
- 1 TEASPOON GROUND FLAXSEED
- 3 ICE CUBES

Makes 1 serving.

Per serving: 265 calories, 17 g protein, 41 g carbohydrates, 5 g total fat (2 g saturated), 136 mg sodium, 7 g fiber

MANGO TANGO

(Number of Powerfoods: 4)

- ½ CUP CUBED MANGO
- ⅓ CUP BLUEBERRIES
- ½ BANANA
- ½ CUP 1 PERCENT MILK
- ½ CUP LOW-FAT VANILLA YOGURT
- 2 TEASPOONS VANILLA WHEY PROTEIN POWDER
- 3 ICE CUBES

Makes 2 servings.

Per serving: 158 calories, 8 g protein, 29 g carbohydrates, 2 g fat (1 g saturated), 80 mg sodium, 2 g fiber

THE IMMUNE BOOSTER

(Number of Powerfoods: 3)

- ½ CUP WATER
- ½ CUP CARROT-APPLE JUICE OR ORANGE JUICE
- 1 SCOOP UNFLAVORED WHEY PROTEIN POWDER
- 1 SCOOP GREEN SUPPLEMENT POWDER (SUCH AS PROGREENS) OR WHEATGRASS POWDER
- 1 TABLESPOON FLAXSEED OIL
- 1 CUP ICE

Makes 1 serving.

Per serving: 360 calories, 27 g protein, 23 g carbohydrates, 15 g fat (2 g saturated), 100 mg sodium, 7 g fiber

ABS DIET POWER TIP

Best late-night snacks for when it's past your bedtime and your stomach's growling like your mother-in-law's lapdog: a small bowl of bran cereal with fat-free milk or a fiber-filled piece of fruit, like a pear. Both snacks contain enough carbs to soothe you into slumber but not enough bulk to make you toss and turn.

SHOW ME THE HONEY
(Number of Powerfoods: 3)

1 SCOOP LOW-FAT BUTTER PECAN
  ICE CREAM
½ CUP 1 PERCENT MILK
1 TABLESPOON VANILLA WHEY
  PROTEIN POWDER
1 TEASPOON GROUND FLAXSEED
  PINCH OF GROUND CINNAMON
1 TEASPOON HONEY
3 ICE CUBES

Makes 1 serving.

Per serving: 250 calories, 15 g protein,
38 g carbohydrates, 4 g fat
(2 g saturated), 131 mg sodium, 3 g fiber

BELLY-BUSTING BERRY
(Number of Powerfoods: 6)

1 SCOOP LOW-FAT VANILLA ICE CREAM
¼ CUP EACH FROZEN BLUEBERRIES,
  STRAWBERRIES, AND RASPBERRIES
½ CUP 1 PERCENT MILK
1 TABLESPOON VANILLA WHEY
  PROTEIN POWDER
3 ICE CUBES

Makes 2 8-ounce servings.

Per serving: 251 calories, 15 g protein,
38 g carbohydrates, 4 g fat
(2 g saturated), 116 mg sodium, 4 g fiber

THE KITCHEN SINK
(Number of Powerfoods: 6)

1 CUP PLAIN YOGURT
1 CUP ICE
¾ CUP FIBER ONE CEREAL
  1 CUP FROZEN BLUEBERRIES
1 SCOOP VANILLA WHEY
  PROTEIN POWDER
1 TABLESPOON GROUND FLAXSEED
1 GENEROUS HANDFUL BABY SPINACH

Makes 2 servings; eat with a spoon.

Per serving: 240 calories, 16 g protein,
39 g carbohydrates, 7 g fat
(4 g saturated), 170 mg sodium, 14 g fiber

CHOCOLATE PUDDING MILK SHAKE

3 CUPS COLD NONFAT MILK
1 PACKAGE (4 SERVINGS)
  JELL-O INSTANT SUGAR-FREE
  CHOCOLATE PUDDING MIX
1½ CUPS VANILLA ICE CREAM

Makes 5 servings.

Per serving: 190 calories, 8 g protein,
31 g carbohydrates, 4.5 g fat
(3 g saturated), 650 mg sodium, 2 g fiber

ABS DIET POWER TIP

Make an extra-quick fruit sorbet. Open a can of peaches, the light-syrup kind, and transfer contents to a large plastic freezer bag. Place the bag in a bowl and put in the freezer overnight. Place the plastic bag of frozen peaches in a pan of hot water for about a minute. Open the bag and pour the liquid into a blender. Transfer the frozen peaches to a cutting board and chop into 1-inch pieces. Then dump into the blender with the syrup, and puree.

BERRY BANANA BUBBLY
(Number of Powerfoods: 1)

1½ CUPS SPARKLING MINERAL WATER
  1 CUP FROZEN STRAWBERRIES, HALVED
  ½ FROZEN BANANA, SLICED

Makes 2 servings.

Per serving: 40 calories, 0 g protein,
10 g carbohydrates, 0 g fat
(0 g saturated), 0 mg sodium, 2 g fiber

THE ENDLESS SUMMER
(Number of Powerfoods: 4)

¼ CUP 1 PERCENT MILK
¾ CUP READY-TO-EAT CUBED SEEDLESS
   WATERMELON PIECES
½ CUP STRAWBERRIES
½ CUP LOW-FAT PLAIN YOGURT
 2 TEASPOONS VANILLA WHEY
   PROTEIN POWDER
 3 ICE CUBES

Makes 1 serving.

Per serving: 110 calories, 8 g protein,
18 g carbohydrates, 1.5 g fat (0.5 g saturated), 60 mg sodium, 1 g fiber

FLOWER POWER
(Number of Powerfoods: 3)

1¼ CUPS FAT-FREE MILK
  ¼ CUP ORANGE JUICE
  ¾ CUP FAT-FREE VANILLA YOGURT
  ⅓ CUP FAT-FREE WHIPPED TOPPING
  ½ CUP FROZEN STRAWBERRIES
  ½ CUP FROZEN CAULIFLOWER FLORETS

Makes 2 servings.

Per serving: 190 calories, 11 g protein,
35 g carbohydrates, 0 g fat
(0 g saturated), 140 mg sodium, 1 g fiber

BEET THE BLUBBER
BLUEBERRY-ALMOND
(Number of Powerfoods: 2)

½ CUP UNSWEETENED CARROT JUICE
¼ CUP FROZEN BLUEBERRIES
¼ CUP PEELED AND GRATED RAW BEET
¼ CUP UNSWEETENED APPLESAUCE
¼ CUP UNSALTED RAW WHOLE ALMONDS
⅓ CUP ICE CUBES
½ TEASPOON FRESH LIME JUICE
 2 GRAMS GLUCOMANNAN
   DASH OF GROUND GINGER

Makes 1 serving.

Per serving: 324 calories, 10 g protein,
35 g carbohydrates, 19 g fat
(1.5 g saturated) 65 mg sodium, 8 g fiber

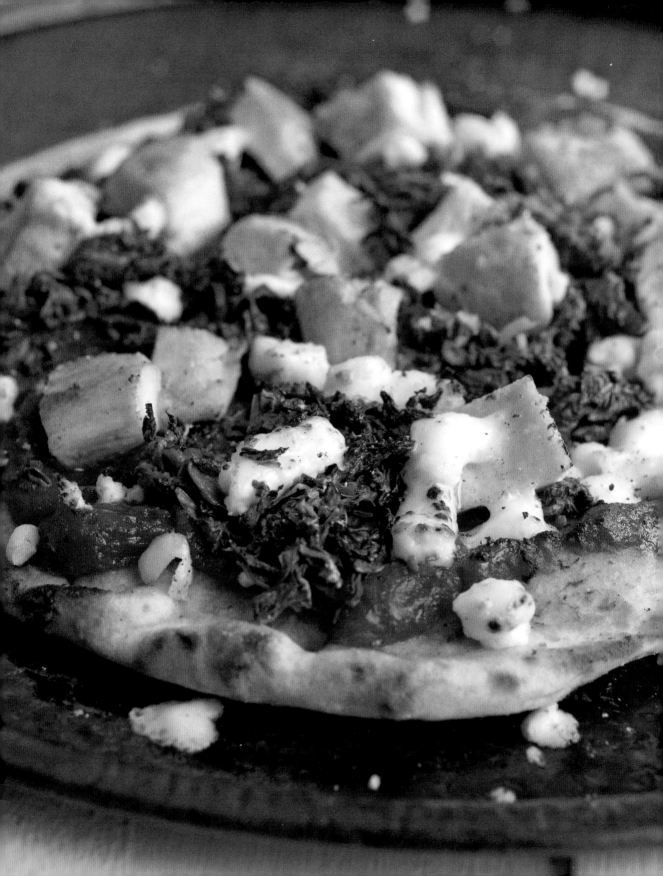

CHICKEN SPINACH PITA PIZZA
(Number of Powerfoods: 4)

3 TABLESPOONS MARINARA SAUCE

1 LARGE PITA OR OTHER FLATBREAD

⅓ CUP FROZEN SPINACH, THAWED AND DRAINED

¼ CUP CRUMBLED FETA CHEESE

¾ CUP CHOPPED COOKED CHICKEN BREAST

SALT AND PEPPER

Spread the marinara sauce over the pita. Top with the spinach, cheese, and chicken. Season with salt and pepper. Bake at 375°F for 6 minutes.

Makes 1 serving.

Per serving: 440 calories, 46 g protein, 33 g carbohydrates, 14 g fat (7 g saturated), 990 mg sodium, 6 g fiber

MEN'S HEALTH SPICY OVEN FRIES
Goes great with The Official Abs Diet Burger, page 195.

4 RUSSET POTATOES,
   CUT LENGTHWISE INTO 12 WEDGES

2 EGG WHITES, LIGHTLY BEATEN

1 TEASPOON CHILI POWDER

1 TEASPOON GROUND CUMIN

1 TEASPOON PAPRIKA

1 TEASPOON DRIED OREGANO

¼ TEASPOON DRIED THYME

1 TEASPOON SALT

⅛ TEASPOON CAYENNE PEPPER

1. Preheat the oven to 450°F. Coat a baking sheet with cooking spray. Dip the cut potatoes in the eggs to coat and place in a bowl. Mix the remaining ingredients and sprinkle over the potatoes; toss well to coat.

2. Place the wedges on the baking sheet. Bake for 20 minutes. Turn the potatoes over and bake for 15 minutes longer or until crisp.

Makes 4 servings.

Per serving: 180 calories, 7 g protein, 40 g carbohydrates, 0.5 g fat (0 g saturated), 640 mg sodium, 4 g fiber

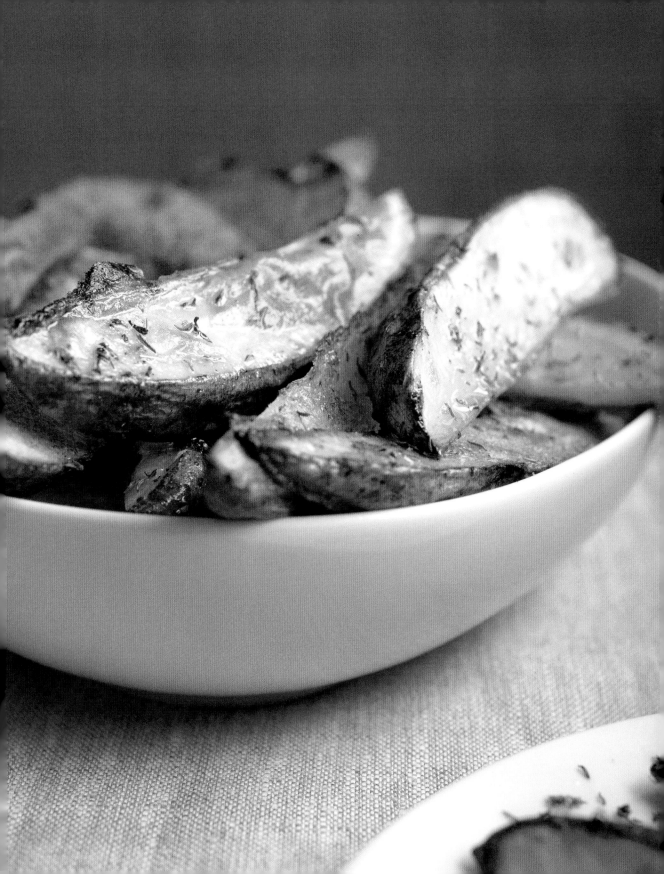

BETTER THAN FRIED CHICKEN FINGERS

Add ketchup instead of soy sauce and kids will think they're fried chicken nuggets; you will, too.
(Number of Powerfoods: 3)

²/₃ CUP LOW-SODIUM SOY SAUCE

6 TABLESPOONS RICE WINE VINEGAR

7 TABLESPOONS WATER

3 SCALLIONS, SLICED

2½ TABLESPOONS SUGAR

1 TABLESPOON GRATED FRESH GINGER

1½ TEASPOONS TOASTED SESAME OIL

½ TEASPOON CRUSHED RED-PEPPER FLAKES

1½ POUNDS BONELESS, SKINLESS CHICKEN BREASTS

2 EGG WHITES

¾ CUP WHOLE GRAIN PASTRY FLOUR

3 TABLESPOONS SESAME SEEDS, TOASTED

1. Combine the soy sauce, vinegar, 6 tablespoons of water, scallions, sugar, ginger, oil, and red-pepper flakes in a medium bowl. Transfer ⅓ cup of the sauce to a large bowl. Cover and refrigerate the remaining sauce.

2. Cut the chicken into ¾-inch-wide strips. Add the chicken to the sauce in the large bowl. Toss well to coat. Allow to marinate for 15 minutes.

3. In a medium bowl, beat the egg whites and remaining 1 tablespoon of water. In another bowl, combine the flour and sesame seeds. Preheat the oven to 350°F. Coat a baking sheet with cooking spray.

4. Dip the chicken strips into the egg mixture and then into the flour mixture, shaking off the excess. Place on a baking sheet. Spray the chicken with cooking spray. Bake for 5 minutes, remove from the oven, and turn the chicken. Spray the other side and bake for 5 minutes longer or until golden brown and cooked through. Serve with the refrigerated soy sauce dip.

Makes 10 servings.

Per serving: 150 calories, 17 g protein, 13 g carbohydrates, 3.5 g fat (0.5 g saturated), 700 mg sodium, 1 g fiber

Fattiest Party Finger Foods

If it's breaded, fried, or swimming in mayo, stay clear.

THE EATS	CALORIES	CARBS (G)	FAT (G)	SAT. FAT (G)
Pigs in blankets (5)	470	33	29	9
Cheese quesadilla (5 ounces)	470	39	26	12
Fried calamari (6 ounces)	350	26	10	4
Fried chicken wings (2)	318	11	21	6
Potato skins (2)	200	18	10	4
Mozzarella sticks (2)	200	16	12	4
Spinach dip (2 tablespoons)	170	1	18	3

SNEAKY GREEK CRUDITÉ DIP

Serve chilled with raw carrots, celery, zucchini, broccoli, cauliflower, and peppers, along with pita wedges or whole wheat crackers.
(Number of Powerfoods: 2)

2 CUPS LOW-FAT PLAIN GREEK YOGURT

1 TABLESPOON DIJON MUSTARD

1 TABLESPOON CHOPPED FRESH DILL

1 CUP BABY SPINACH LEAVES, CHOPPED

½ CUP SEEDED, GRATED CUCUMBER

1 CLOVE GARLIC, MINCED

1 TEASPOON LEMON JUICE

Whisk the ingredients in a bowl until smooth. Chill.

Makes 4 servings.

Per serving: 70 calories, 9 g protein, 6 g carbohydrates, 2 g fat (1.5 g saturated), 130 mg sodium, 0 g fiber

HUMMUS A TUNA

For a change, try substituting 1 tablespoon light mayonnaise for the hummus and adding 1 tablespoon sweet pickle relish and ½ teaspoon Old Bay seasoning. Spoon the tuna mixture onto two or three Bibb lettuce leaves.
(Number of Powerfoods: 3)

1 CAN (3 OUNCES) SOLID WHITE TUNA IN WATER, DRAINED AND FLAKED

2 HEAPING TABLESPOONS HUMMUS (CHICKPEA SPREAD)

1 TEASPOON LEMON JUICE

2 WASA CRISPBREAD CRACKERS

Mix the tuna, hummus, and lemon juice in a bowl. Spoon onto the crackers.

Makes 1 serving.

Per serving: 250 calories, 25 g protein, 26 g carbohydrates, 6 g fat (1 g saturated), 520 mg sodium, 6 g fiber

Leanest Party Finger Foods

These appetizers will satisfy your hunger without overloading you with calories.

THE EATS	CALORIES	CARBS (G)	FAT (G)	SAT. FAT (G)
Salsa (2 tablespoons)	9	2	0.1	0
Popcorn (handful, no butter)	31	6	0.4	0.1
Grapes (handful)	34	4	0.1	0
Hummus (2 tablespoons)	46	4	3	0.4
Brie (0.6 ounce)	57	0.1	5	3
Shrimp (3 ounces)	84	0	1	0.2
Edamame (2 ounces)	85	8	3	0.5
California roll (4 pieces)	130	19	4	0.5
Chicken kebab (6 ounces)	150	4	2	0

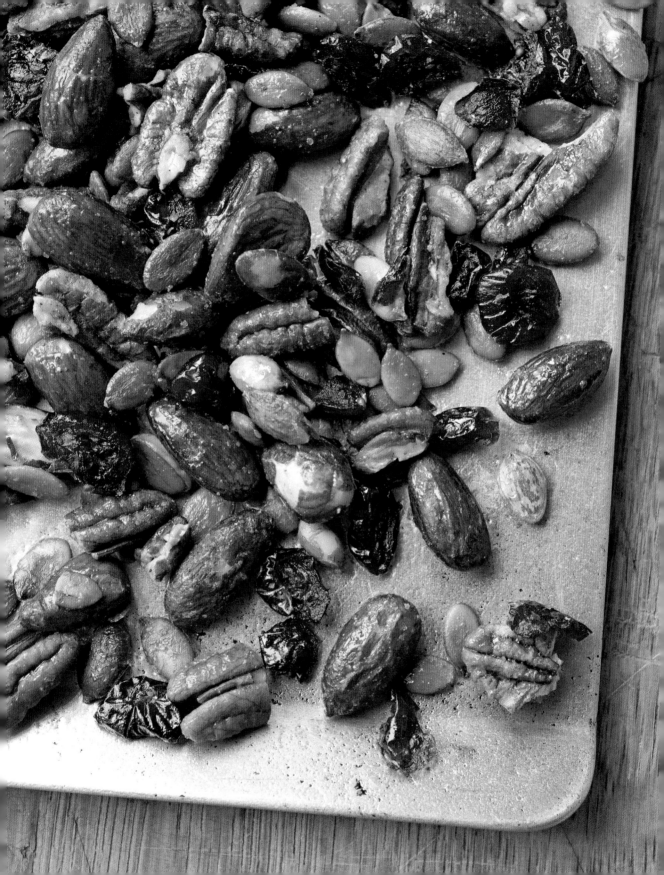

TAILGATE PARTY NUT MIX

Serve at parties or place servings into resealable bags to stash at work or in the car.
(Number of Powerfoods: 4)

1 CUP PUMPKIN SEEDS

1 TEASPOON CANOLA OIL

1 CUP WHOLE ALMONDS

1 CUP PECAN HALVES

2 TABLESPOONS MAPLE SYRUP

½ TEASPOON GROUND CINNAMON

½ TEASPOON GROUND NUTMEG

½ TEASPOON GROUND ALLSPICE

½ TEASPOON SEA SALT

1 CUP ORANGE-FLAVORED
　 DRIED CRANBERRIES

1. Preheat the oven to 350°F. Coat a baking sheet with cooking spray. Put the pumpkin seeds in a bowl and coat with the oil. Spread the seeds on the baking sheet and roast for about 20 minutes, stirring several times.

2. Place the pumpkin seeds, almonds, and pecans in a medium bowl and stir in the maple syrup to coat. Mix the cinnamon, nutmeg, allspice, and salt in a small bowl. Add to the nuts and stir well.

3. Spread the mixture on the baking sheet and roast for 15 minutes, stirring occasionally, until dry. Check often to avoid burning. Cool in the pan for 20 minutes.

4. Place the mix in a bowl and stir in the cranberries.

Makes 12 ¼-cup servings.

Per serving: 260 calories, 7 g protein, 16 g carbohydrates, 20 g fat (2 g saturated), 105 mg sodium, 3 g fiber

ABS DIET POWER TIP

Fresh out of pecan halves? Then switch-hit with walnuts or shelled pistachios. Both may do a number on your LDL (bad) cholesterol. A recent report from Penn State University researchers found that one or two servings of nuts a day can lower LDL cholesterol by up to 12 percent. The magic likely comes from the heart-healthy monoun-saturated fats, phytosterols, and fiber in the nuts.

ABS DIET HALL OF FAME
RIP-ROARIN' ROASTED RED PEPPER SAUCE

Serve with homemade whole wheat pita wedges: Cut each pita into 8 wedges, separate the layers, and spread on a baking sheet. Mist with cooking spray and bake at 350°F for 15 minutes, until crisp.
(Number of Powerfoods: 3)

1 JAR (7 OUNCES) ROASTED RED
    PEPPERS, DRAINED AND CHOPPED
2 TABLESPOONS CHOPPED BASIL
2 TABLESPOONS CHOPPED WALNUTS
1 CLOVE GARLIC, CRUSHED
1 TEASPOON BALSAMIC VINEGAR
1 TABLESPOON EXTRA-VIRGIN OLIVE OIL
    SALT AND PEPPER

Mix the ingredients in a blender or food processor, seasoning with salt and pepper. Process until smooth.

Makes 16 1-tablespoon servings.

Per serving: 23 calories, 0 g protein, 1 g carbohydrates, 2 g fat (0 g saturated), 45 mg sodium, 0 g fiber

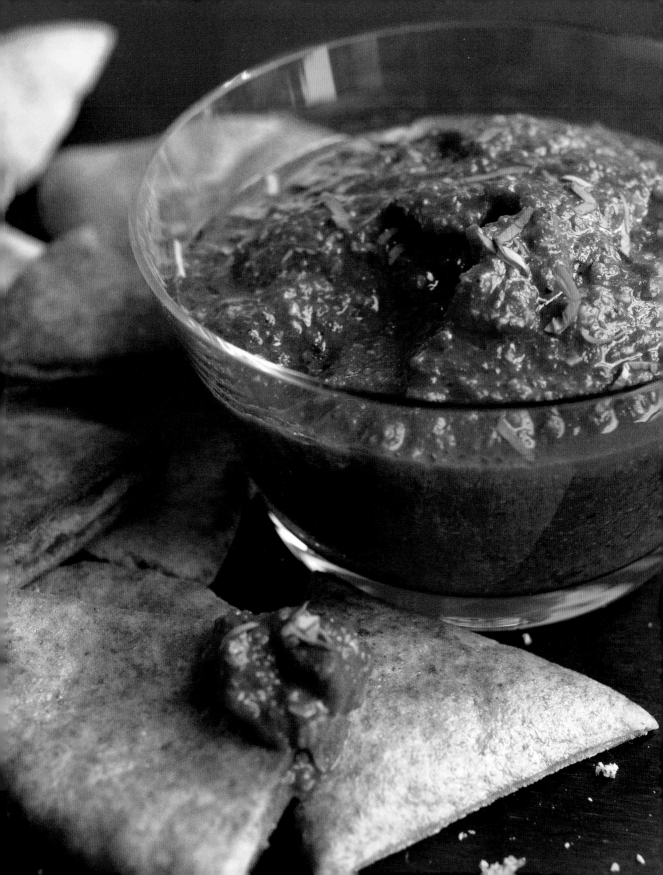

MUFFIN-TO-IT PERSONAL PIZZAS
(Number of Powerfoods: 3)

2 WHOLE GRAIN ENGLISH MUFFINS, SPLIT
¼ CUP PIZZA SAUCE
1 CUP SHREDDED PART-SKIM
  MOZZARELLA CHEESE
8 SLICES TURKEY PEPPERONI

Preheat the oven to 275°F. Place the muffin halves, cut side up, on a baking sheet. Spoon pizza sauce onto each one, spreading with the back of the spoon. Add the cheese and pepperoni slices. Bake for 7 to 10 minutes or until the cheese is melted and a bit browned.

Makes 2 servings.

Per serving: 330 calories, 21 g protein, 30 g carbohydrates, 15 g fat (8 g saturated), 780 mg sodium, 5 g fiber

PIZZA ROLL-UPS
(Number of Powerfoods: 4)

2 TEASPOONS EXTRA-VIRGIN OLIVE OIL
½ MEDIUM ONION, DICED
1 CUP SMALL BUTTON MUSHROOMS, SLICED
½ CUP PIZZA SAUCE
1 LARGE WHOLE WHEAT TORTILLA
¼ CUP SHREDDED PART-SKIM
  MOZZARELLA CHEESE
2 OUNCES LOW-FAT TURKEY
  PEPPERONI SLICES
2 TABLESPOONS GRATED
  PARMESAN CHEESE

1. Heat the oil in a skillet over medium heat. Add the onion and mushrooms and cook for 3 minutes or until the onion is soft.

2. Microwave the pizza sauce, stirring once, until warm, about 90 seconds. Spread the sauce evenly over the tortilla. Spoon on the mushroom mixture, mozzarella, pepperoni, and Parmesan. Fold the outer edges in, then roll. Cut in half.

Makes 2 servings.

Per serving: 270 calories, 19 g protein, 22 g carbohydrates, 13 g fat (4.5 g saturated), 900 mg sodium, 4 g fiber

The Snack Pack 10 mini-meals under 300 calories

1. Stick of string cheese (80)

2. 5 cups light microwave popcorn sprinkled with Old Bay and 1 tablespoon Romano cheese (150)

3. 6 strawberries dipped in yogurt and drizzled with chocolate sauce (150)

4. Clif bar (250)

5. 1 serving (1 ounce) baked tortilla chips with 1 heaping tablespoon guacamole (290)

6. 1 can (3 ounces) tuna with hot sauce on whole grain crackers (160)

7. 1 cup reduced-fat cottage cheese with peaches and cinnamon (200)

8. 2 handfuls black olives (200)

9. 1 egg on a whole grain English muffin with melted cheese (250)

10. 1 cup blackberries or blueberries with 6 ounces light yogurt and 1 tablespoon low-fat granola (200)

ABS DIET HALL OF FAME
GUILTLESS TAILGATE WINGS
(Number of Powerfoods: 2)

3 TABLESPOONS HOT SAUCE

2 TABLESPOONS LOW-SODIUM
   WORCESTERSHIRE SAUCE

1 TABLESPOON HONEY

½ TEASPOON PAPRIKA

1 CLOVE GARLIC, CRUSHED

12 BONELESS, SKINLESS CHICKEN
   TENDERS (ABOUT 12 OUNCES)

2 TABLESPOONS LOW-FAT
   BLUE CHEESE DRESSING

1. Mix the hot sauce, Worcestershire, honey, paprika, and garlic in a large bowl. (If the honey clumps, nuke the mixture for 10 to 15 seconds and then stir.) Place the chicken and half of the sauce in a large resealable bag. Close and shake to coat each piece.

2. Heat a large skillet over medium heat. Remove the chicken from the bag and cook for 1 to 2 minutes on each side; discard any sauce left in the bag. Add the chicken to the bowl with the remaining sauce mixture and toss to coat. Serve with the dressing.

Makes 2 servings.

Per serving: 250 calories, 35 g protein, 14 g carbohydrates, 5 g fat (1 g saturated), 800 mg sodium, 1 g fiber

TAKE A QUICK DIP
(Number of Powerfoods: 2)

1 CAN (15 OUNCES) CANNELLINI BEANS,
   RINSED AND DRAINED

1 TABLESPOON CHOPPED FRESH
   ROSEMARY

1 CLOVE GARLIC, CRUSHED

½ LEMON, JUICED

2 TABLESPOONS OLIVE OIL
   SALT AND PEPPER TO TASTE

In a blender or food processor, puree the beans, rosemary, garlic, and lemon juice. Stream oil through the top until you reach the desired consistency. Season to taste with salt and pepper.

Per 1-tablespoon serving: 21 calories, 1 g protein, 2 g carbohydrates, 1 g fat (0 g saturated), 20 mg sodium, 1 g fiber

DILL-ICIOUS DIP
(Number of Abs Diet Powerfoods: 3)

1 CUP LOW-FAT PLAIN YOGURT

⅓ CUP DICED CUCUMBER

¼ CUP DICED ONION

⅓ TEASPOON DILL

Stir ingredients together in a small bowl until well blended.

Makes 1 serving.

Per 1-tablespoon serving: 10 calories, 1 g protein, 1 g carbohydrate, 0 g fat (0 g saturated), 9 mg sodium, 0 g fiber

FIT FACT

Eating protein after a workout speeds fat loss. In a British study, men who ate a snack high in protein (43 grams) and low in carbohydrates burned 21 percent more fat than men who chugged a sugary recovery drink. What's magical about protein? It requires more energy to process in your gut than carbs do.

LITTLE DRUMMERS, BOY

These buffalo chicken drummettes have more meat than wings and baked
without their skin brings the calories and fat way down.
(Number of Powerfoods: 2)

24 CHICKEN DRUMMETTES, SKINNED
 4 TABLESPOONS HOT SAUCE
 5 TEASPOONS WHITE WINE VINEGAR
 2 TABLESPOONS HONEY
 ¼ TEASPOON GARLIC POWDER
 ⅓ CUP CRUMBLED BLUE CHEESE
 1 CUP SOUR CREAM
 1 SCALLION, CHOPPED
 2 LARGE RIBS CELERY, CUT INTO STICKS
 ½ TEASPOON PAPRIKA

1. Remove as much of the skin from the chicken as you can. In a large bowl, toss the drummettes with the hot sauce, vinegar, honey, and garlic powder, until each piece is well-coated. Refrigerate for at least an hour.

2. Arrange the drummettes on the rack of a broiler pan. Broil 5 inches from the heat for about 20 minutes, or until the meat is no longer pink and is cooked through, turning once.

3. To make the blue cheese dip, combine the blue cheese, sour cream, and scallion. Mix well. Then sprinkle with paprika. Cover and refrigerator for 20 minutes or until the flavors blend. Serve dressing with chicken drummettes and celery sticks.

Makes 12 2-wing servings.

Per serving: 120 calories, 14 g protein, 2 g carbohydrates, 6 g fat (2.5 g saturated), 240 mg sodium, 0 g fiber

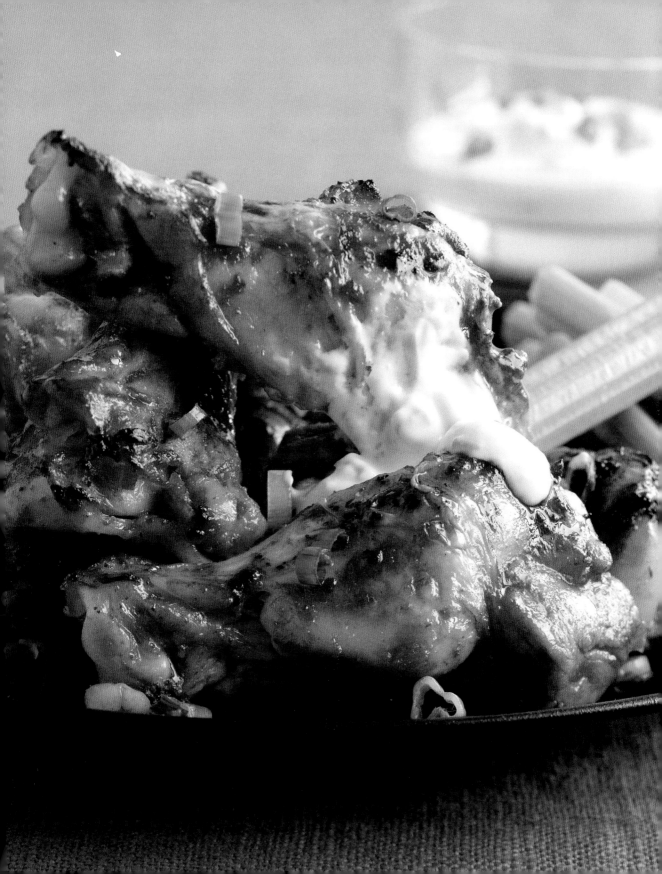

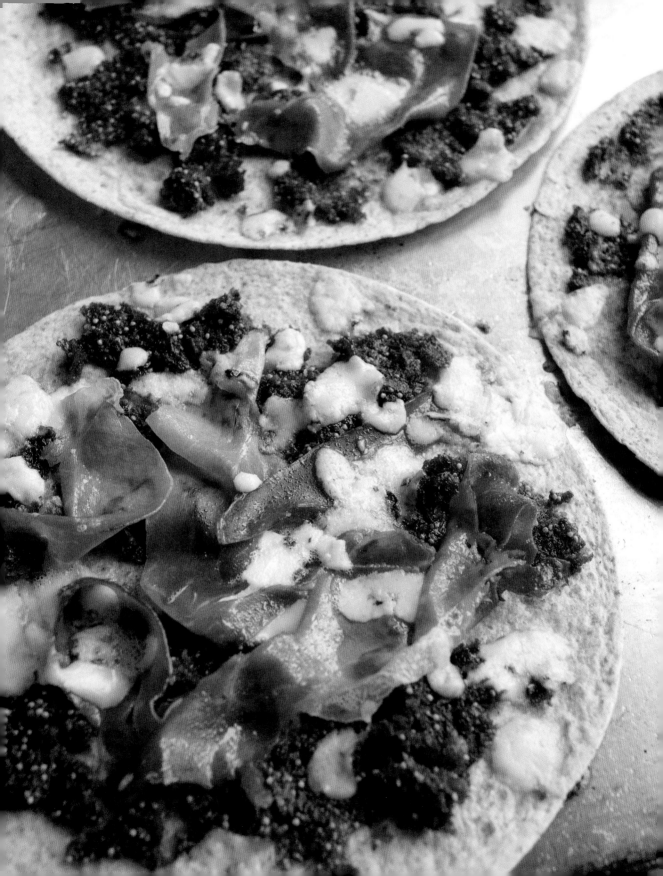

FIG AND PROSCIUTTO TORTILLA BITES

A sweet and savory appetizer that'll impress your guest(s).
(Number of Powerfoods: 3)

1 16-OUNCE PACKAGE FIGS,
   STEMMED, HALVED
4 6-INCH WHOLE GRAIN TORTILLAS
¼ POUND PROSCIUTTO HAM
4 OUNCES GORGONZOLA CHEESE

1. Place the figs in a saucepan filled with 1 cup of water over medium heat; cover. Simmer for 5 minutes, then remove from the heat. Preheat an oven to 350°F.

2. After the figs have cooled (about 10 minutes), puree in a blender for 2 minutes. Coat a skillet with nonstick spray. Toast one tortilla at a time over medium-high heat.

3. Spread 2 tablespoons of the pureed figs over the toasted tortillas. Top each with 2 slices of prosciutto and 1½ tablespoons gorgonzola. Place the tortillas on a baking sheet and bake on the center rack for 10 minutes or until the cheese melts and the prosciutto becomes crisp. Cut into wedges.

Makes 8 servings (half a "pizza" each).

Per serving: 150 calories, 7 g protein, 22 g carbohydrates, 5 g fat (3 g saturated), 430 mg sodium, 3 g fiber

CHAPTER 6

The New Abs Diet Lunches

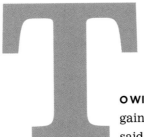

O WIN THE WAR AGAINST weight gain, remember what Napoleon said: An army travels on its stomach. If you can't control the food lines, you can't win the war.

That's what makes lunch the most hazardous meal of the day. It's the meal that's most out of our control, the one that too often comes via chain restaurant, fast-food court, or vending machine. (Or, if we're among the lucky few, it comes from a thick, juicy expense account.) And therein lies the danger, my friends: Want a filling, delicious sandwich? You could stop by Quiznos, but their Prime Rib Cheesesteak Sub effectively delivers 1,070 calories—almost half of what you should eat in an entire day—in about 12 bites. Rather go Mexican? On the Border's Grande Taco Salad with Taco Beef weighs in at 1,620 calories—enough calories to pack on nearly half a pound of flab in one sitting! Too freaked out by the food and figure you'll just have a soft drink? Jeez, don't go ordering one of "The Hulk" drinks at Smoothie King: A strawberry smoothie will cost you a whopping 2,088 calories—about the equivalent of FIVE Wendy's quarter-pound burgers.

Now, it's not my intention to freak you out: Counting calories is no way to enjoy a corned beef on pumpernickel rye. But it pays to occasionally glance at the calorie and fat gram numbers in fast food, if only to remind yourself how dangerous lunchtime in America can be for someone trying to lose weight.

To get a more accurate and personal picture, try this little experiment: Keep a food diary for two days in which you patronize a coffee shop, deli, or restaurant at least once. Record what you eat and how much. List everything that goes in your mouth—drinks and snacks, too. Then grab a calorie book or jump on the Internet and find the calories in the foods and beverages on your list. Tally up your numbers; I think you'll be surprised, even shocked by the number of calories you consumed. Regular restaurant eating will make it difficult to make a dent in your belly. Remember the lesson of the USDA study that found that people who frequent fast-food restaurants consume, on average, 500 more calories a day than people who make meals at home.

Ah, but you can save the couple of bucks a day—and the 130,000 calories a year—by preparing your own lunch. I know, I know—brown-bagging it can seem like a hassle. You have to remember to make it, you have to remember to bring it, and you have to not spill it along the way. Chicken soup may be good for the soul, but it doesn't hold up so well when you're being jostled in a commuter train or trying to keep your lunch from hitting the windshield in stop-and-go traffic. So, you need to think about portability and plan ahead, at least on workdays.

The easy solution: Make lunch while you're making dinner. You're already in the kitchen, and you've got to do something with yourself while you're waiting for the pasta to boil. There are plenty of ways to whip up a fast and portable lunch in this chapter, as well as genius ideas for turning last night's leftovers into tomorrow's treat. (Hint: Keep whole wheat tortillas and pita pockets on hand for wrapping and filling quick lunches.) So don't give in to the tyranny of the fast-food lunch every day. You don't have to.

Here's how to start taking back control!

Quick Lunches Tip

You can trim your carbohydrate and calorie intake in sandwiches by nearly 50 percent by choosing the right kind of bread loaves at the supermarket. Buy the soft-style or thin-cut breads that typically weigh less than 30 grams per slice. Also, try to select whole wheat bread that contains at least 3 grams of fiber per slice. Cheese? Choose provolone, which has more calcium, slightly fewer calories, and less saturated fat than most other cheeses.

Turn the page for 25 New Abs Diet–approved recipes!

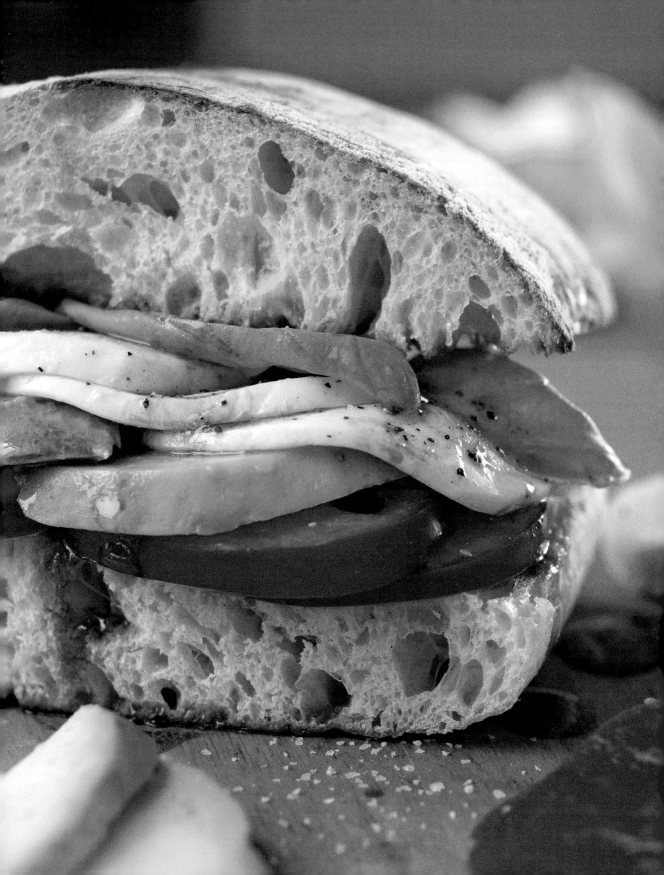

THE TOM BOY
(Tomato, AvocadO, Mozzarella, Basil)
(Number of Powerfoods: 3)

1 LOAF ITALIAN OR
   CIABATTA BREAD

6 FRESH BASIL LEAVES

2 LARGE TOMATOES, SLICED

1 AVOCADO, PITTED, PEELED, AND SLICED

4 OUNCES FRESH MOZZARELLA
   CHEESE, SLICED

3 TABLESPOONS EXTRA-VIRGIN
   OLIVE OIL

1 TABLESPOON BALSAMIC VINEGAR
   SEA SALT AND CRACKED BLACK PEPPER

1. Slice the bread in half lengthwise and toast both halves. Layer the basil, tomato slices, avocado, and cheese evenly on half of the bread.

2. Mix the oil and vinegar in a small bowl and drizzle on top of the sandwich. Sprinkle with salt and pepper and top with the remaining bread half. Cut into slices.

Makes 2 servings.

Per serving: 510 calories, 17 g protein, 24 g carbohydrates, 42 g fat (10 g saturated), 180 mg sodium, 7 g fiber

---

ABS DIET HALL OF FAME **POPEYE AND OLIVE OIL SALAD**
(Number of Powerfoods: 4)

FOR THE SALAD:

1½ CUPS CHOPPED BABY SPINACH

1½ CUPS CHOPPED ROMAINE LETTUCE

3 SLICES PROSCIUTTO, CHOPPED

½ CUP MANDARIN ORANGE SLICES

⅓ CUP SLICED STRAWBERRIES

2 TABLESPOONS DICED RED ONION

FOR THE DRESSING:

1½ TEASPOONS EXTRA-VIRGIN OLIVE OIL

1 TABLESPOON RED WINE VINEGAR

½ CLOVE GARLIC, MINCED

⅛ TEASPOON BLACK PEPPER

Mix the salad ingredients in a bowl. Mix the dressing in another bowl and pour over the salad. Toss to coat.

Makes 1 serving.

Per serving: 238 calories, 9 g protein, 23 g carbohydrates, 14 g fat (4 g saturated), 450 mg sodium, 6 g fiber

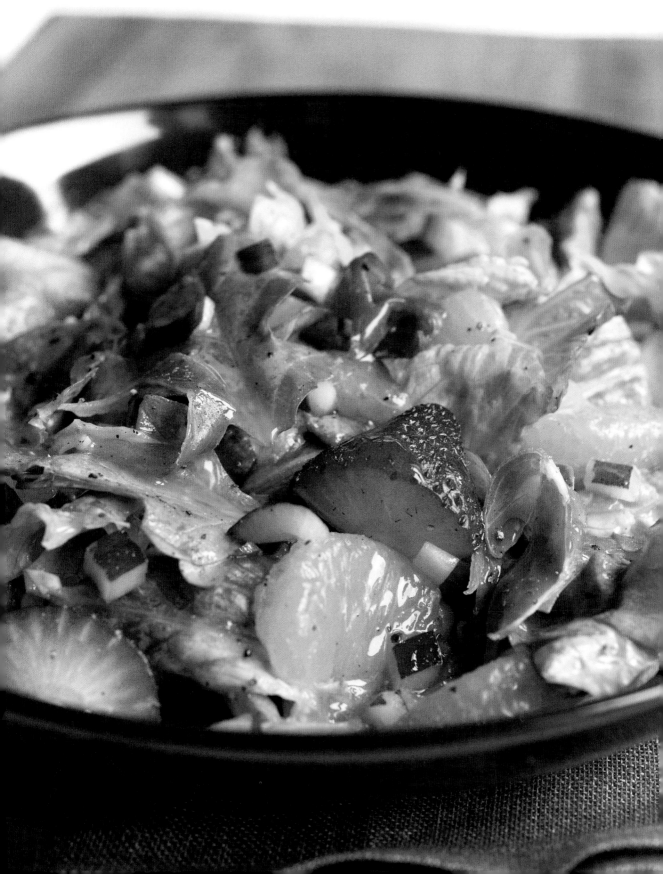

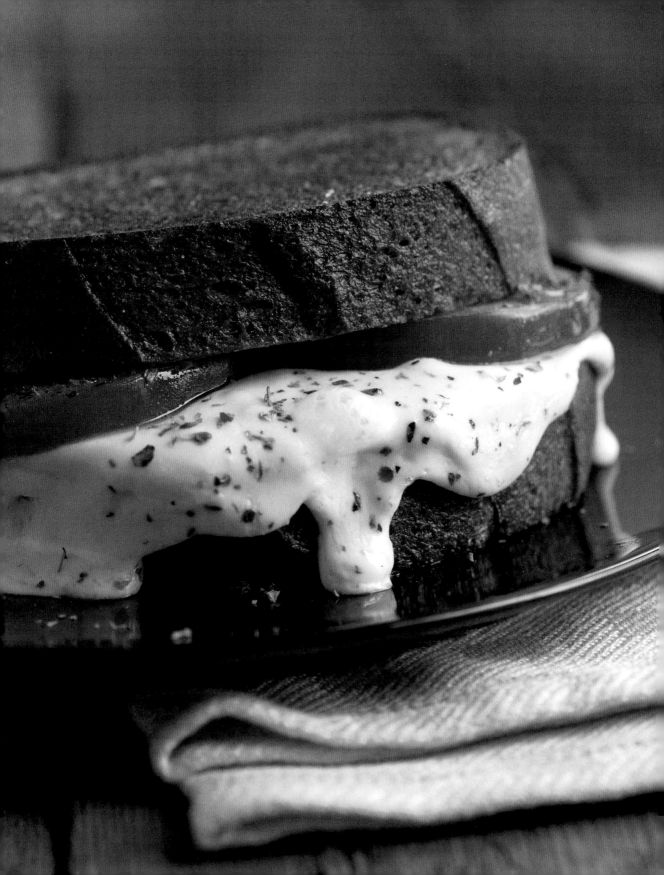

GROWN-UP GRILLED CHEESE
We grew up on Velveeta grilled cheese sandwiches.
This version cuts the fat in half and dumps the white bread.
(Number of Powerfoods: 3)

1 TEASPOON OLIVE OIL
2 SLICES (OR ½ CUP) PART-SKIM
   MOZZARELLA CHEESE
2 SLICES TOMATO
2 SLICES WHOLE WHEAT BREAD
   OREGANO TO TASTE

Add the oil to a skillet and place over
medium heat. Slip the cheese and
tomato slices onto a slice of bread.
Sprinkle oregano on top. Cover with the
second bread slice. Grill the sandwich
until the cheese melts.

Makes 1 serving.

Per serving: 330 calories, 21 g protein,
26 g carbohydrates, 15 g fat
(7 g saturated), 35 mg sodium, 4 g fiber

TEQUILA SUNRISE SALAD
(Number of Powerfoods: 5)

FOR THE SALAD:

2½ CUPS MIXED GREENS
¼ CUP BLACK BEANS,
   RINSED AND DRAINED
1 PLUM TOMATO, CHOPPED
1 SCALLION, SLICED
½ AVOCADO, PEELED AND SLICED
1 TEASPOON CHOPPED CILANTRO

FOR THE DRESSING:

1 TABLESPOON TEQUILA
1 TABLESPOON ORANGE JUICE
1 TEASPOON LIME JUICE
1 TEASPOON EXTRA-VIRGIN OLIVE OIL
   CRACKED BLACK PEPPER

Mix the salad ingredients in a bowl. Mix the dressing in another bowl and pour over the salad. Toss to coat.

Makes 1 serving.

Per serving: 325 calories, 8 g protein, 22 g carbohydrates, 21 g fat (3 g saturated), 250 mg sodium, 13 g fiber

CHIPOTLE MAYONNAISE

1 CUP LIGHT MAYONNAISE
1 TABLESPOON SEEDED AND FINELY
   CHOPPED CANNED CHIPOTLE CHILES
2 TEASPOONS ADOBO SAUCE (FROM CAN)
¼ TEASPOON LEMON JUICE

Whisk the ingredients together in a small bowl. Refrigerate until ready to use.

Makes 16 1-tablespoon servings.

Per serving: 50 calories, 0 g protein, 1 g carbohydrate, 5 g fat (1 g saturated), 250 mg sodium, 0 g fiber

THE THANKSGIVING DAY-AFTER PARTY
(Number of Powerfoods: 4)

2 TABLESPOONS CRANBERRY RELISH
1 WHOLE WHEAT TORTILLA
3 SLICES LEFTOVER CARVED TURKEY
1 SLICE MUENSTER CHEESE
¾ CUP MIXED GREENS

Spread the cranberry relish down the center of the tortilla. Add turkey and remaining ingredients. Fold outer edges in, then roll.

Makes 1 serving.

Per serving: 311 calories, 24 g protein, 40 g carbohydrates, 11 g fat (6 g saturated), 1,063 mg sodium, 3 g fiber

EAT-THE-BOWL BEAN SALSA
(Number of Powerfoods: 2)

1 CAN (15 OUNCES) BLACK BEANS,
   RINSED AND DRAINED
2 MEDIUM TOMATOES, DICED
2 TABLESPOONS FROZEN
   ORANGE JUICE CONCENTRATE
½ CUP CHOPPED CILANTRO
   SALT
2 LARGE RED BELL PEPPERS

1. Mix the beans, tomatoes, orange juice concentrate, and cilantro in a bowl. Season with salt. Refrigerate for 30 minutes to allow the flavors to blend.

2. Slice the top off the peppers and scoop out the core and seeds. Fill with the bean mixture.

Makes a little more than 2 servings.

Per serving: 280 calories, 15 g protein, 49 g carbohydrates, 2.5 g fat (0 g saturated), 670 mg sodium, 16 g fiber

ABS DIET POWER TIP

Use hummus (made from chickpeas) as a sandwich condiment. It packs a load of fiber and mayonnaise-like richness without a ton of calories. Try it with roast beef and roasted red peppers.

MEXI-CALI TUNA SALAD
(Number of Powerfoods: 3)

1 CAN (3 OUNCES) CHUNK LIGHT TUNA
IN WATER, DRAINED
¾ CUP CANNED BLACK BEANS,
RINSED AND DRAINED
½ CUP SALSA
½ RIPE AVOCADO, PEELED AND CHOPPED

Mix the tuna, beans, and salsa in
a bowl. Top with the avocado.

Makes 1 serving.

Per serving: 460 calories, 36 g protein,
42 g carbohydrates, 17 g fat (2.5 g saturated), 1,660 mg sodium, 19 g fiber

THE JOHNNY APPLE
CHEESE SANDWICH
(Number of Powerfoods: 3)

2 SLICES 7-GRAIN BREAD
2 TEASPOONS LIGHT MAYONNAISE
1 TEASPOON DIJON MUSTARD
2 SLICES SWISS CHEESE
1 RED DELICIOUS APPLE, HALVED,
CORED, AND THINLY SLICED
1 TABLESPOON CHOPPED WALNUTS

1. Preheat a toaster oven to 350°F.

2. Spread 1 bread slice with mayonnaise
and the other with mustard. Top each
with cheese.

3. Place on a tray and put into the
toaster oven until the cheese has
melted. Top 1 slice with the apple slices
and sprinkle with the walnuts.
Press the sandwich halves together.

Makes 1 serving.

Per serving: 440 calories, 19 g protein,
46 g carbohydrates, 21 g fat
(7 g saturated), 500 mg sodium, 8 g fiber

ROAST BEEF AND
HORSERADISH WRAP
(Number of Powerfoods: 3)

2 TEASPOONS LIGHT MAYONNAISE
½ TEASPOON PREPARED HORSERADISH
1 WHOLE WHEAT TORTILLA
1 LARGE ROMAINE LETTUCE LEAF
3 SLICES LEAN ROAST BEEF
¼ CUP CHOPPED TOMATO

1. Mix the mayonnaise and horseradish
in a small bowl. Spread the mixture on
one side of the tortilla.

2. Place the lettuce leaf in the center of the
tortilla, followed by the roast beef and
tomato. Fold the outer edges in, then roll.

Makes 1 serving.

Per serving: 190 calories, 17 g protein,
23 g carbohydrates, 6 g fat
(1.5 g saturated), 640 mg sodium, 3 g fiber

THAI-THAI BIRDIE
(Number of Powerfoods: 4)

1 WHOLE WHEAT TORTILLA
1½ TABLESPOONS CHUNKY
PEANUT BUTTER
⅔ CUP CHOPPED COOKED CHICKEN
¼ CUP MATCHSTICK CARROTS
¾ CUP MIXED GREENS
1 TEASPOON CHOPPED CILANTRO
1 TEASPOON CHILI SAUCE

Warm the tortilla according to the
package directions. Spread peanut
butter down the center and add the
chicken and remaining ingredients.
Fold the outer edges in, then roll.

Makes 1 serving.

Per serving: 390 calories, 39 g protein,
31 g carbohydrates, 16 g fat
(3 g saturated), 470 mg sodium, 6 g fiber

**ABS DIET
POWER TIP**

Try broccoli
sprouts instead
of lettuce on your
next turkey sand-
wich. The sprouts
are rich in sulfo-
raphane, a phyto-
chemical that
studies have
shown can stifle
the H. pylori gut
bacteria that
causes ulcers.

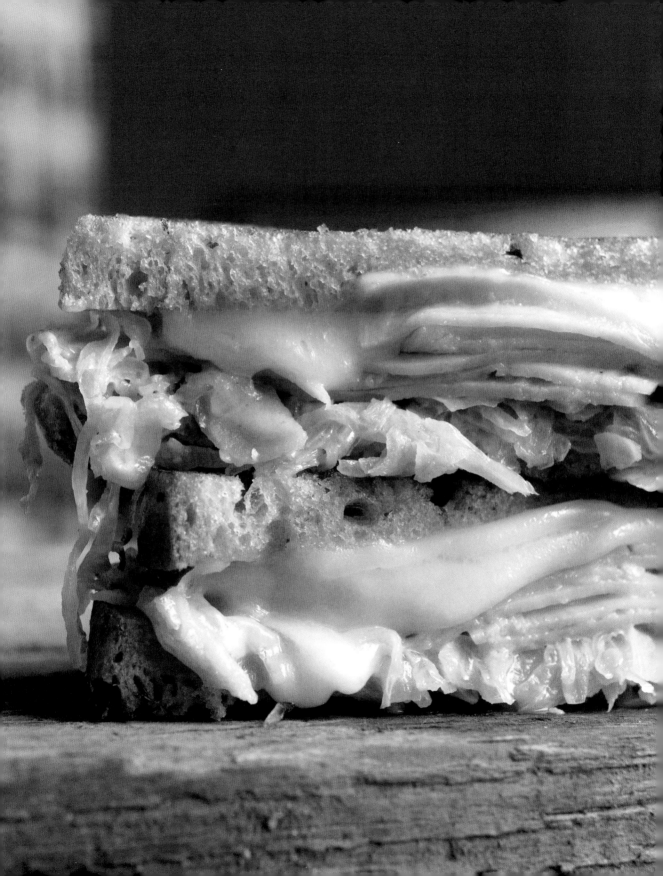

REUBEN MADE BETTA
(Number of Powerfoods: 3)

¼ CUP CANNED SAUERKRAUT,
   RINSED TWICE AND DRAINED WELL

1 TABLESPOON CRUMBLED FETA CHEESE

1 TABLESPOON LOW-FAT THOUSAND
   ISLAND DRESSING

2 SLICES RYE BREAD

2 SLICES REDUCED-SODIUM SMOKED
   DELI TURKEY

1 SLICE LOW-FAT SWISS OR
   MOZZARELLA CHEESE

1. Mix the sauerkraut, feta, and dressing in a small bowl. Spread on 1 bread slice. Top with the turkey, cheese, and the remaining bread.

2. Coat a nonstick skillet with cooking spray and place over medium heat until hot. Add the sandwich and grill for 2 to 3 minutes per side until the cheese has melted.

Makes 1 serving.

Per serving: 335 calories, 23 g protein, 42 g carbohydrates, 9 g fat (3 g saturated), 1,625 mg sodium, 5 g fiber

THE MUSCLE MAKER
(Number of Powerfoods: 3)

1 PLUM TOMATO, CUT INTO EIGHTHS
¼ CUP SLICED ONION
1 SMALL CLOVE GARLIC, CRUSHED
2½ CUPS CHOPPED ROMAINE LETTUCE
2 TABLESPOONS BALSAMIC VINAIGRETTE
  SALT AND PEPPER
  GRILLED FLANK STEAK SLICES
2 TABLESPOONS CRUMBLED
  BLUE CHEESE

1. Mix the tomato, onion, garlic, and lettuce in a bowl. Add the vinaigrette and toss to coat. Season with salt and pepper.

2. Top with the steak and cheese.

Makes 1 serving.

Per serving: 350 calories, 38 g protein, 16 g carbohydrates, 16 g fat (7 g saturated), 680 mg sodium, 4 g fiber

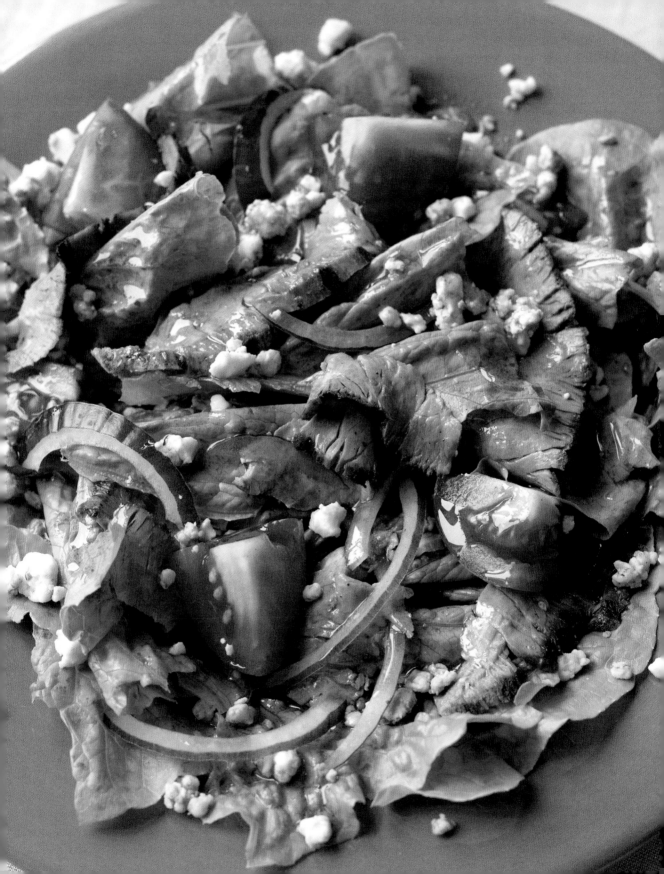

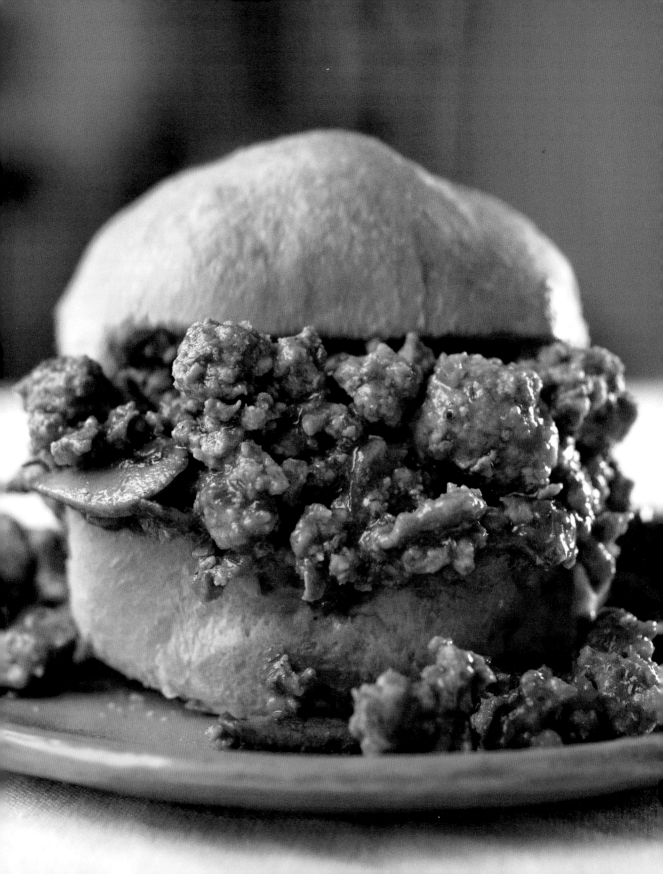

VERY SLOPPY JOES WITH 'SHROOMS
(Number of Powerfoods: 2)

1½ POUNDS LEAN GROUND TURKEY
¼ POUND MUSHROOMS, SLICED
½ TEASPOON GARLIC POWDER
1 CUP KETCHUP
¼ CUP APPLE CIDER VINEGAR
2 TABLESPOONS YELLOW MUSTARD
½ TABLESPOON CHILI POWDER
¼ CUP WORCESTERSHIRE SAUCE
GROUND BLACK PEPPER
4 WHOLE WHEAT HAMBURGER BUNS

1. Coat a large skillet with cooking spray and place over medium heat until hot. Add the turkey and mushrooms; cook for 3 minutes, stirring to break up the meat. Add the garlic powder. Reduce the heat to low and cook for 3 minutes.

2. Stir in the ketchup, vinegar, mustard, chili powder, and Worcestershire. Continue cooking over low heat for 5 to 10 minutes, stirring occasionally.

3. Season with pepper. Spoon the mixture over the bun bottoms and add the tops.

Makes 4 servings.

Per serving: 460 calories, 40 g protein, 38 g carbohydrates, 18 g fat (4 g saturated), 1,357 mg sodium, 7 g fiber

DON'T TELL MOM IT'S NOT MEAT LOAF

Make this turkey meat loaf for dinner, then slice up the leftovers for cold sandwiches, slathered with ketchup, for lunch. For a spicier condiment, try chipotle mayonnaise (page 132).
(Number of Powerfoods: 2)

2 CUPS DICED ONIONS
2 TABLESPOONS EXTRA-VIRGIN OLIVE OIL
2½ POUNDS GROUND LEAN TURKEY
2 EGGS
3 TABLESPOONS CHOPPED CILANTRO
1 TABLESPOON MINCED GARLIC
2 TEASPOONS GROUND CUMIN
2 CUPS DICED TOMATOES
  SALT AND PEPPER
1 CUP MARINARA SAUCE

1. Preheat the oven to 350°F. Coat two 9-by-5-inch loaf pans with cooking spray.

2. Heat a large nonstick skillet over medium heat until hot. Cook the onions in the oil until lightly browned. Let cool, transfer to a bowl, and mix in the turkey, eggs, cilantro, garlic, cumin, tomatoes, and salt and pepper. Divide between the prepared pans.

3. Spread the sauce on top. Loosely cover with foil and bake for 45 minutes or until cooked through.

Makes 8 servings.

Per serving: 310 calories, 28 g protein, 9 g carbohydrates, 18 g fat (4 g saturated), 280 mg sodium, 2 g fiber

QUESADILLA AL ROMA

A good use for leftover rotisserie chicken and sautéed vegetables.
(Number of Powerfoods: 3)

1 TABLESPOON SUN-DRIED TOMATO PESTO
1 WHOLE WHEAT TORTILLA
½ CUP SHREDDED PART-SKIM MOZZARELLA CHEESE
½ CUP CHOPPED COOKED CHICKEN
1 CUP SAUTÉED ONIONS, RED BELL PEPPERS, AND MUSHROOMS

Spread the pesto on the tortilla. Top with the cheese, chicken, and vegetables. Microwave open-faced for 1 minute or until the cheese has melted. Fold in half and slice into wedges.

Makes 1 serving.

Per serving: 400 calories, 40 g protein, 31 g carbohydrates, 15 g fat (7 g saturated), 740 mg sodium, 4 g fiber

GO FIG-URE PANINI
(Number of Powerfoods: 4)

- 1 CIABATTA ROLL
- 4 THIN SLICES HAM
- 2 SLICES SWISS CHEESE
- 2 FRESH FIGS, SLICED
- 1 SMALL HANDFUL ARUGULA

1. Split the roll and layer the bottom half with 2 ham slices, the cheese, figs, arugula, and the remaining ham.

2. Top with the other half of the roll and heat in a panini press until the cheese melts.

Makes 1 serving.

Per serving: 490 calories, 32 g protein, 43 g carbohydrates, 22 g fat (12 g saturated), 890 mg sodium, 4 g fiber

DRINK THIS
THE ABS DIET ARNOLD PALMER
For a light summer evening cocktail, stir in 1 cup spiced dark rum.

- 7 CUPS WATER
- 2 BLACK TEA BAGS
- 1 CUP LOOSELY PACKED FRESH MINT LEAVES
- 1 CAN (6 OUNCES) FROZEN LEMONADE CONCENTRATE, THAWED
- 1 LIME, SLICED
- 1 LEMON, SLICED
- 1 ORANGE, SLICED

1. Boil 3 cups of the water. Pour into a teapot and add the tea bags and mint. Steep for 10 minutes.

2. Strain the tea into a 3-quart container. Stir in the remaining 4 cups water and lemonade concentrate. Add slices of lime, lemon, and orange as garnish. Serve in tall glasses over ice.

Makes 9 servings.

Per serving: 15 calories, 0 g protein, 5 g carbohydrates, 0 g fat, (0 g saturated), 5 mg sodium, 0 g fiber

ABS DIET POWER TIP

Order unsweetened iced tea instead of soda. A 20-ounce sugary soft drink contains upward of 17 teaspoons of sugar and 255 calories. A gallon of unsweetened iced tea? Zero. Bonus: Tea delivers more antioxidants than does a serving of carrots or broccoli.

BUFFALO MEATBALL SANDWICH

Ground buffalo makes this meatball sandwich low in fat and rich in flavor.
(Number of Powerfoods: 5)

1 POUND LEAN GROUND BUFFALO

2 EGG WHITES

½ CUP TOASTED WHEAT GERM

⅓ CUP FINELY CHOPPED ONION

2 TABLESPOONS GRATED PARMESAN CHEESE

1 TEASPOON MINCED GARLIC

1 FRENCH BAGUETTE OR CRUSTY ITALIAN BREAD

1 TABLESPOON EXTRA-VIRGIN OLIVE OIL

½ TEASPOON SALT-FREE ALL-PURPOSE SEASONING

¼ TEASPOON BLACK PEPPER

1 JAR (14 OUNCES) SPAGHETTI SAUCE

4 THIN SLICES MOZZARELLA CHEESE

1. Preheat the oven to 350°F.

2. Mix the buffalo, egg whites, wheat germ, onion, Parmesan, and garlic. Shape into 12 meatballs and place in a baking dish that's been lightly coated with cooking spray. Bake for 15 to 20 minutes (turning once) or until cooked through.

3. While the meatballs are cooking, slice the baguette in half lengthwise and remove some of the interior bread to trim the carbs and make room for the meatballs. With 5 minutes left to bake the meatballs, place the bread in the oven to lightly toast. Brush the meatballs with the oil and season with the all-purpose seasoning and pepper.

4. Warm the spaghetti sauce in a pan over medium heat. Spoon the meatballs into the sauce to coat and then line them up in the bottom bread half. Top with the mozzarella.

5. Return the baguette to the oven for about 2 minutes or until the cheese melts. Allow to cool for a minute and cut into slices.

Makes 4 servings.

Per serving: 580 calories, 46 g protein, 54 g carbohydrates, 19 g fat (7 g saturated), 1,120 mg sodium, 5 g fiber

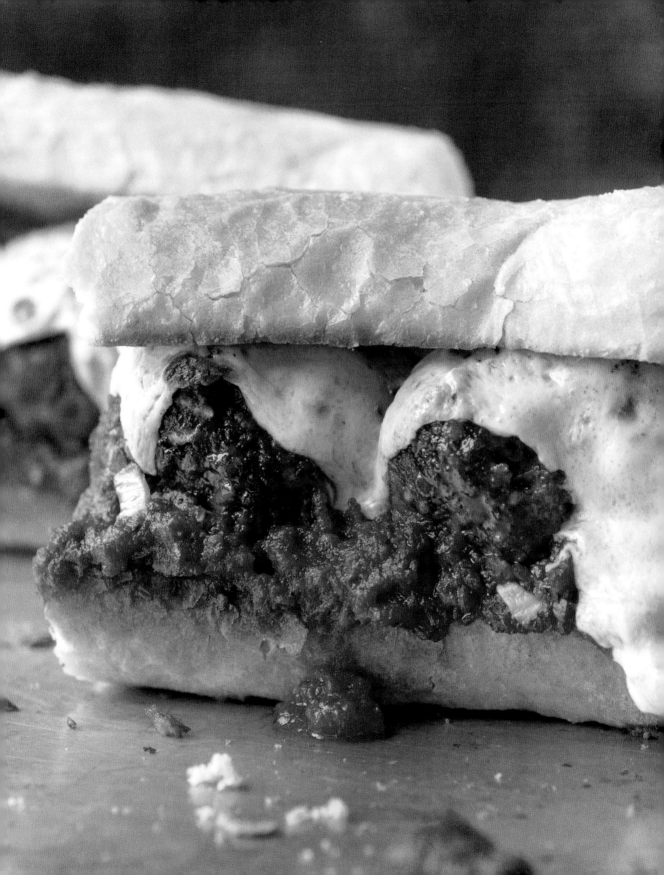

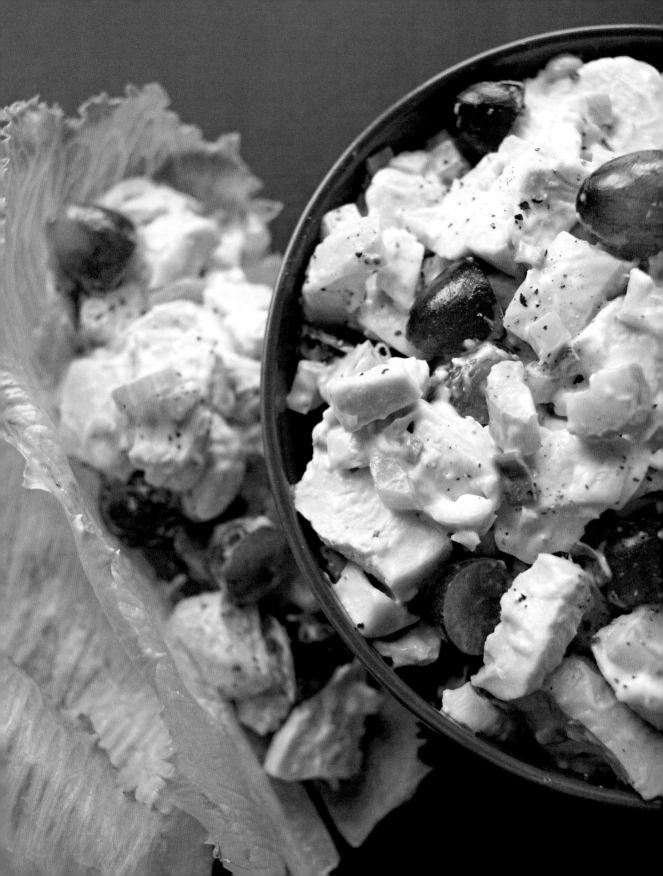

MAN-CAN-LIVE-WITHOUT-BREAD CHICKEN SALAD SANDWICH
(Number of Powerfoods: 2)

2 COOKED CHICKEN BREASTS, CHOPPED

½ CUP CHOPPED CELERY

½ SCALLION, CHOPPED

2 TABLESPOONS LIGHT MAYONNAISE

    SALT AND PEPPER

½ CUP HALVED SEEDLESS RED GRAPES

2 ROMAINE OR RED LEAF
    LETTUCE LEAVES

1. Mix the chicken, celery, scallion, and mayonnaise in a bowl; season with salt and pepper. Gently stir in the grapes.

2. Divide between the lettuce leaves and roll up.

Makes 2 servings.

Per serving: 230 calories, 27 g protein, 10 g carbohydrates, 8 g fat (1.5 g saturated), 200 mg sodium, 1 g fiber

NIGHT-BEFORE THAI NOODLES
(Number of Powerfoods: 2)

½ POUND WHOLE WHEAT FETTUCCINE
1 TABLESPOON TOASTED SESAME OIL
2 CUPS SNOW PEAS
½ MEDIUM RED PEPPER,
    SLICED INTO MATCHSTICKS
2 GRILLED CHICKEN BREASTS, CHOPPED

FOR THE DRESSING:
3 TABLESPOONS SOY SAUCE
½ TABLESPOON PEANUT OIL
2 TABLESPOONS TOASTED SESAME OIL
2 TEASPOONS RICE VINEGAR
1 TABLESPOON SUGAR
2 SCALLIONS, THINLY SLICED
1 TABLESPOON GRATED FRESH GINGER
1 CLOVE GARLIC, MINCED
3 TEASPOONS MONGOLIAN FIRE OIL

1. Mix the dressing ingredients in a bowl.

2. Cook the fettuccine following the directions on the package. Drain well. Place in a large bowl, add the sesame oil, toss to coat, and refrigerate until cold, at least 15 minutes.

3. Cook the snow peas in boiling water for 1 minute, drain, and cool. Add the peas and pepper to the pasta.

4. Stir the dressing to combine, pour over the pasta, and toss to coat. Top with the chicken. Serve cold.

Makes 4 servings.

Per serving: 330 calories, 20 g protein, 27 g carbohydrates, 17 g fat (3 g saturated), 790 mg sodium, 5 g fiber

BEAN THERE, DONE THAT
(Number of Powerfoods: 3)

1½ CANS (15 OUNCES EACH) BLACK BEANS,
    RINSED AND DRAINED
½ CUP CHICKEN BROTH
1 CHOPPED PLUM TOMATO
1 SCALLION, SLICED
1 TABLESPOON LIME JUICE
1 TEASPOON HOT SAUCE
1 TEASPOON EXTRA-VIRGIN OLIVE OIL
1 TABLESPOON CHOPPED CILANTRO
½ TEASPOON GROUND CUMIN
    SALT AND PEPPER
1 TABLESPOON SHREDDED REDUCED-FAT
    MEXICAN-BLEND CHEESE

Dump everything except the cheese into the blender. Process until smooth, scraping the sides as needed. Pour into bowls and microwave for 2 or 3 minutes, stirring occasionally. Sprinkle with cheese.

Makes 4 servings.

Per serving: 365 calories, 24 g protein, 60 g carbohydrates, 5 g fat (1 g saturated), 475 mg sodium, 22 g fiber

THE CLUBMAN
(Number of Powerfoods: 5)

2 SLICES WHOLE WHEAT BREAD
2 SLICES REDUCED-SODIUM SMOKED
  TURKEY
2 GREEN LEAF LETTUCE OR SPINACH
  LEAVES
1 SLICE PROVOLONE CHEESE
½ AVOCADO, SLICED

Toast the bread and top with the rest of the ingredients. You won't need mayonnaise. The avocado will moisten the sandwich nicely.

Makes 1 serving.

Per serving: 410 calories, 22 g protein, 41 g carbohydrates, 22 g fat (5 g saturated), 1,148 mg sodium, 11 g fiber

EGG YOURSELF ON
(Number of Powerfoods: 5)

1 EGG
2 SLICES WHOLE WHEAT BREAD
2 SLICES REDUCED-SODIUM DELI HAM
1 SLICE LOW-FAT CHEDDAR CHEESE
1 SLICE TOMATO
2 LEAVES ROMAINE LETTUCE

1. Lightly coat a nonstick skillet with cooking spray and add egg. Fry to desired doneness.

2. While cooking the egg, toast the bread. Add the ham, cheese, tomato, and lettuce (in that order) to one slice of toast. Top with the hot egg and remaining bread slice.

Makes 1 serving.

Per serving: 331 calories, 28 g protein, 30 g carbohydrates, 11 g total fat (4 g saturated), 950 mg sodium, 4 g fiber

PACO'S FISH TACOS
(Number of Powerfoods: 5)

2 CUPS RED CABBAGE, THINLY SLICED
4 SCALLIONS, THINLY SLICED
½ CUP REDUCED-FAT SOUR CREAM
2 TABLESPOONS FRESH LIME JUICE
½ JALAPEÑO CHILE PEPPER, MINCED
1 TABLESPOON TACO SEASONING
1 TABLESPOON OLIVE OIL
1 POUND TILAPIA FILLETS (OR OTHER
  WHITE FISH), CUT INTO 16 STRIPS
  SALT AND PEPPER TO TASTE
8 WHOLE WHEAT TORTILLAS
  (8-INCH DIAMETER)
½ CUP FRESH CILANTRO LEAVES
8 LIME WEDGES

1. In a large bowl, combine cabbage, scallions, taco seasoning, sour cream, lime juice, and minced jalapeño.

2. Pour the olive oil in a large non-stick skillet and swirl to coat the bottom of the pan. Warm the oil over medium-high heat, then add the fish, seasoned on both sides with salt and pepper. Cook the fish for about 6 minutes on all sides until golden brown. (If there's too much fish for one skillet, cook two batches.)

3. Warm the tortillas. Fill each tortilla with the slaw mixture, then add the fish and cilantro leaves. Fold in half. Serve with lime wedges.

Makes 4 serving.

Per serving: 490 calories, 31 g protein, 54 g carbohydrates, 5 g fat (2 g saturated), 750 mg sodium, 5 g fiber

ABS DIET POWER TIP

When there's no time to brown-bag your workday lunch and fast food is your only option, build your own healthier "sandwich" at the drive-through. Order a plain grilled chicken sandwich and a baked potato with sour cream. Eat the potato flesh and leave the skin. Toss the white-bread buns (to save calories) and tuck the chicken breast inside the potato skin. (That's where all the nutrients and fiber are found.) Top with salsa and eat like a sandwich.

CHAPTER 7

The New Abs Diet Soups, Salads, and Side Dishes

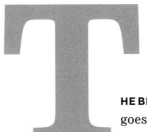

HE BEST DEFENSE, as the saying goes, is a good offense, not only on the football field, the battle-field, or in personal finance, but especially at the supper table.

For example, let's say you're quarterbacking tonight's meal and the menu is showing blitz. You've got three meatballs the size of linebackers inching toward you behind a mountain of your favorite spaghetti with sauce. And to your blindside is a monstrous defensive end, a loaf of garlic bread named Carb Overload.

They're coming for you. What are you going to do?

Your first thought: portion control. Even the healthiest meal can get sacked by second helpings and tackled by thirds. But how do you stay in control, especially when the food's so darn good?

Fortunately, you have the best offensive linemen in the league up front—your soup and salad—skilled blockers to defend against the rush of hunger. By preparing for the food blitz with high-volume, low-calorie appetizers and a smattering of protein, you can avoid being trampled by your main course. Consider:

■ A Penn State study found that people who ate soup before an entrée reduced their total calorie intake by 20 percent compared with people who did not eat soup before the meal. Low-calorie, broth-based soups fill your belly quickly, triggering signals to your brain that say, "Hey, everything's cool; we're not starving anymore."

■ A salad made with vegetables and protein provides a double dose of protection against overeating. Protein stifles hunger. Crunchy vegetables consist mostly of water and fiber, which fill you up and slow digestion at the expense of very few calories. Try a French salade niçoise made with eggs, tuna, chickpeas, and all the vegetables you want. It delivers 42 grams of muscle-building, hunger-busting protein, as much as in a New York strip steak.

■ Elevating side dishes to entrée status is one of the most effective ways to lose weight. Who says the meat and potatoes have to take center stage? Treat the meat or pasta as a side dish, taking up a quarter to a third of your plate, and make the vegetables your main meal. In one study, when people swapped half the roast beef and rice on their plates with lightly buttered broccoli, they ate 86 fewer calories at the meal and felt just as satisfied. The fiber in that broccoli probably had something to do with it. Just like the liquid in soup, fiber creates a sense of fullness in the stomach. What's more, fiber slows the absorption of sugars, which dampens your hunger. Want to get more fiber from your broccoli, cauliflower, and carrots? Steam them before eating them. Heat makes fiber more available, so you'll get up to twice the amount of fiber that you'd get by eating those vegetables raw. For a terrific side dish to turn into a main meal, try Wok the Broc, page 171.

■ In addition to soups, salads, and sides, even a small piece of bread dipped in extra-virgin olive oil can help you control overeating your main meal. The monounsaturated fat in that tasty appetizer is satiating. Not only that, compounds in olive oil may stimulate the function of mitochondria, the "power plants" of the cells in our bodies, preventing obesity and diabetes, according to new research published in the *Journal of Nutritional Biochemistry*.

The Abs Diet works so effectively because it utilizes study-based strategies like these to outwit your hunger. If you build a blockade of soups, salads, and side dishes into your meal plan, you won't have to worry much about calorie counting and portion sizes. The threat of that loaf of garlic bread will be easily neutralized. And you'll be too busy enjoying the delicious meals to recognize how healthfully you're eating.

Quick Soups, Salads, and Side Dishes Tip

An unusual side dish can turn a mundane chicken breast into a gourmet-quality meal. Pick up fennel at your grocer or farmers market. This crunchy, sweet, aromatic vegetable with a mild licorice flavor is loaded with vitamin C and other antioxidants. Here's how to cook it: Cut off the core at the base of the bulb and remove the long stems. Quarter the bulb and saute it with a teaspoon of olive oil in a pan over medium heat. After 5 minutes, lower the heat and add $1/2$ cup of orange juice. Cover and simmer until the fennel is soft, about 10 minutes. (Hey, fennel is also great grilled. Just brush with olive oil before tossing on a hot grill.)

Turn the page for 28 New Abs Diet–approved recipes!

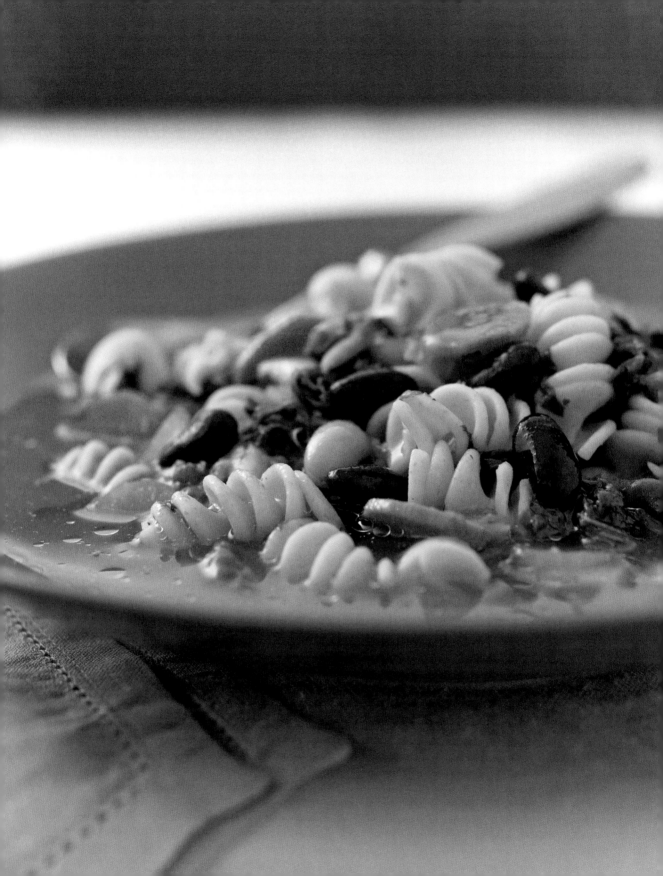

SLOW COOKER RECIPE **DUMP-AND-GO MINESTRONE**
(Number of Powerfoods: 5)

2 TABLESPOONS EXTRA-VIRGIN OLIVE OIL

2 CANS (16 OUNCES EACH) LOW-SODIUM CHICKEN BROTH

1 CAN (15.5 OUNCES) CANNELLINI BEANS, RINSED AND DRAINED

1 CAN (15 OUNCES) RED KIDNEY BEANS, RINSED AND DRAINED

2 CANS (14.5 OUNCES) DICED TOMATOES

5 LARGE CARROTS, THINLY SLICED

1 CUP DICED CELERY

2 CLOVES GARLIC, CHOPPED

1 LARGE ONION, DICED

½ TEASPOON DRIED OREGANO

½ TEASPOON BLACK PEPPER

1 PACKAGE WHOLE WHEAT ROTINI OR SIMILAR PASTA

1 PACKAGE (10 OUNCES) FROZEN SPINACH, THAWED AND SQUEEZED DRY

1. Dump all of the ingredients, except the pasta and spinach, into a large slow cooker. Stir to mix. Cover and cook on low for 6 to 8 hours.

2. Cook the pasta according to the package directions. Add the pasta and spinach to the cooker and stir. Turn up to high and cook for 10 minutes.

Makes 10 servings.

Per serving: 247 calories, 7 g protein, 46 g carbohydrates, 1 g fat (0.5 g saturated), 364 mg sodium, 8 g fiber

FOOD FACT

You can unleash more alliinase, a heart-healthy compound in garlic, by allowing freshly chopped garlic to rest for 10 minutes before cooking, according to Argentine researchers.

ALL 'CHOKED UP
For a zestier flavor, try peppery arugula instead of spinach.
(Number of Powerfoods: 3)

4 CUPS BABY SPINACH

1 CAN (14 OUNCES) ARTICHOKE HEARTS
  IN WATER, DRAINED

1 CAN (15 OUNCES) CANELLINI BEANS,
  RINSED AND DRAINED

1 CUP GRAPE TOMATOES, HALVED

1 JAR (7 OUNCES) ROASTED RED PEPPERS

2 TABLESPOONS EXTRA-VIRGIN
  OLIVE OIL

¼ CUP LEMON JUICE

1 TABLESPOON WATER

½ TEASPOON DRIED OREGANO
  GROUND BLACK PEPPER TO TASTE

1. Wash and shake the water off the spinach. Place 1 cup on each salad plate. Cut the drained artichoke hearts vertically into quarters. Then divide the beans, artichoke hearts, and tomatoes evenly on top of the spinach on each plate. Slice the roasted peppers into finger-thick strips and add to the salads.

2. For the dressing, whisk the oil, lemon juice, water, oregano, and pepper in a small bowl. Using a spoon, drizzle over each salad.

Makes 4 servings.

Per serving: 230 calories, 9 g protein, 33 g carbohydrates, 8 g fat (1 g saturated), 1,540 mg sodium, 10 g fiber

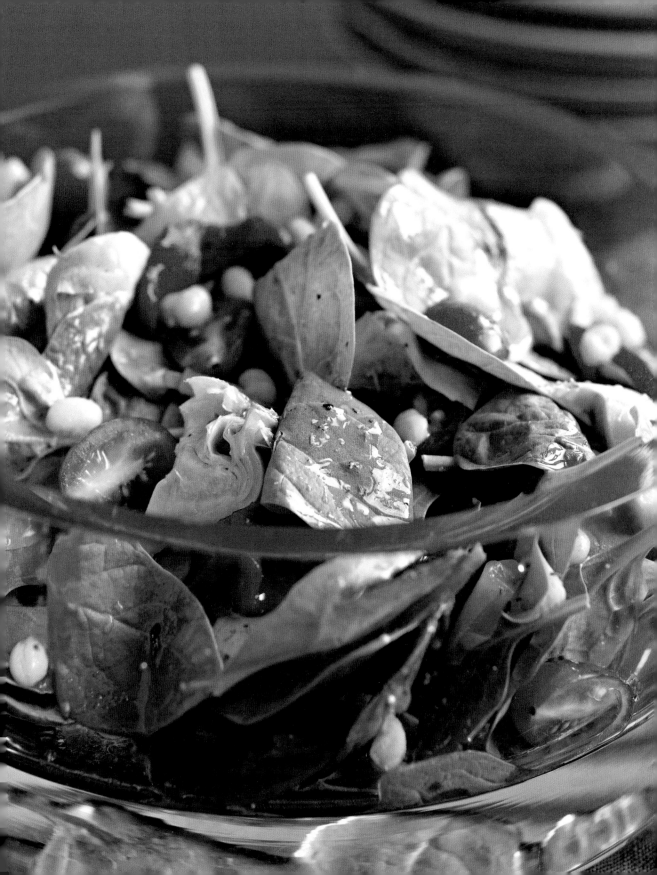

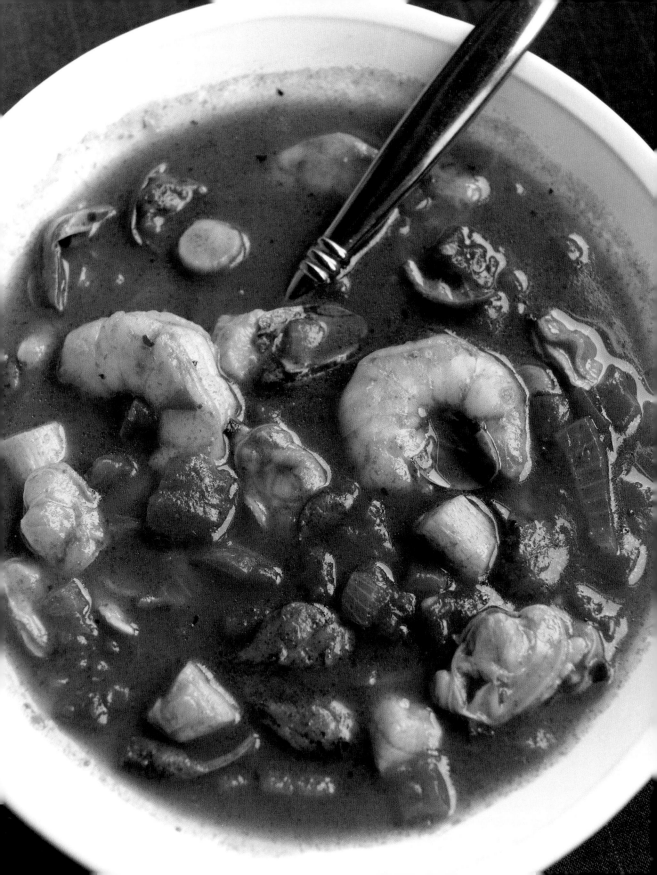

GREETINGS FROM ASBURY PARK SEAFOOD STEW
(Number of Powerfoods: 3)

1 TABLESPOON OLIVE OIL
½ CUP CHOPPED ONION
½ CUP CHOPPED RED BELL PEPPER
1 CLOVE GARLIC, MINCED
1 CAN (28 OUNCES) DICED TOMATOES
1 CAN (28 OUNCES) TOMATO SAUCE
¼ CUP DRY RED WINE
¼ CUP CHOPPED PARSLEY
1 TEASPOON WORCESTERSHIRE SAUCE
½ TEASPOON DRIED OREGANO
1 TEASPOON RED-PEPPER FLAKES
8 OUNCES BAY SCALLOPS
8 OUNCES MEDIUM SHRIMP,
  PEELED AND DEVEINED
1 CAN (10 OUNCES) WHOLE CLAMS
1 PACKAGE BABY SPINACH

1. Heat the oil in a Dutch oven or large pot over medium-high heat. Add the onion, bell pepper, and garlic. Sauté for 5 minutes or until the onion is tender.

2. Dump in the tomatoes (with juice), tomato sauce, wine, parsley, Worcestershire, oregano, and pepper flakes. Stir well. Bring to a boil over medium heat and then simmer, covered, for 20 minutes, stirring occasionally.

3. Add the scallops, shrimp, and clams. Bring to a boil; reduce the heat. Stir. Simmer for 8 minutes or until the scallops are tender and the shrimp turn pink. During the last minute of cooking, add the baby spinach.

Makes 6 servings.

Per serving: 288 calories, 37 g protein, 22 g carbohydrates, 5 g fat (1 g saturated), 1,380 mg sodium, 4.5 g fiber

FIT FACT

Most people who lose weight and maintain the loss share four common behaviors:

90% exercise every day.

78% eat a healthy breakfast every day.

75% weigh themselves at least once a week.

62% watch fewer than 10 hours of TV per week.

Source: Data from the National Weight Control Registry

BEAN TO FLORIDA? SALAD
(Number of Powerfoods: 3)

2 FLORIDA NAVEL ORANGES

½ RED ONION

1 CAN (14.5 OUNCES) CHICKPEAS, RINSED AND DRAINED

1 CAN (14.5 OUNCES) RED KIDNEY BEANS, RINSED AND DRAINED

¼ CUP REDUCED-FAT ITALIAN SALAD DRESSING

1 TABLESPOON EXTRA-VIRGIN OLIVE OIL

1 TABLESPOON BALSAMIC VINEGAR

½ TEASPOON BLACK PEPPER

1. Grate the zest of half of 1 orange into a large bowl. Peel the oranges, cut crosswise into slices, and halve the slices; add to the bowl. Cut the onion crosswise into slices and halve the slices; add to the bowl. Stir in the beans.

2. Whisk the dressing, oil, vinegar, and pepper in a small bowl. Pour over the salad and toss to coat.

Makes 6 servings.

Per serving: 119 calories, 5 g protein, 20 g carbohydrates, 4 g fat (0.9 g saturated), 301 mg sodium, 4 g fiber

SOUL-FRIED COLLARDS
(Number of Powerfoods: 2)

1 POUND COLLARD GREENS

½ CUP WATER

¼ CUP EXTRA-VIRGIN OLIVE OIL

1 POUND CABBAGE, THINLY SLICED

1 LARGE CARROT, SHREDDED

2 TABLESPOONS CHOPPED ONION

⅓ CUP SUGAR

1 TABLESPOON RED WINE VINEGAR

1 TEASPOON SALT

1 TEASPOON BLACK PEPPER

HOT SAUCE

1. Wash the collard greens well and squeeze to drain. Dab with paper towels to remove excess water. Cut the stems from the greens. Chop the leaves into 2-inch pieces.

2. Bring the water to a boil in a large pot, add the greens, and return to a boil. Cover, reduce the heat, and simmer for 5 minutes. Drain in a colander.

3. Heat the oil in a large skillet over medium-high heat. Dump in the cabbage, carrot, and onion; stir-fry for 2 minutes. Add the collard greens, sugar, vinegar, salt, and pepper. Stir-fry for 3 minutes. Cover. Reduce the heat and simmer for 5 minutes or until the greens are tender. Season with hot sauce.

Makes 8 servings.

Per serving: 130 calories, 2 g protein, 16 g carbohydrates, 7 g fat (1 g saturated), 370 mg sodium, 4 g fiber

ABS DIET POWER TIP

Collard greens, kale, spinach, and other green leafy vegetables are mental medicine. A study of 3,000 people age 65 and older found that those who ate two servings of vegetables a day had a 40 percent lower rate of cognitive decline than those who ate one serving or less. The likely reason: All those green vegetables are rich in vitamin E. Toss your greens with olive oil to get the biggest benefit. Fat helps your body better absorb vitamin E.

BRAZILIAN RICE AND BEANS
(Number of Powerfoods: 3)

2 TABLESPOONS OLIVE OIL

1 CUP CHOPPED ONION

1 TABLESPOON MINCED GARLIC

1½ TEASPOONS GROUND CUMIN

¼ TEASPOON SALT

¼ CUP CHOPPED BACON

3 CUPS CANNED BLACK BEANS OR RED KIDNEY BEANS, RINSED AND DRAINED

1 CUP LOW-SODIUM CHICKEN BROTH

2 CUPS COOKED INSTANT BROWN RICE

Mix the oil, onion, garlic, cumin, salt, and bacon in a large saucepan. Cook over medium heat, stirring occasionally, for 4 minutes or until the onion is softened. Stir in the beans to coat with the seasonings. Add the broth. Reduce the heat to medium-low. Cover and cook for 15 minutes for the flavors to blend. Serve over the rice.

Makes 4 servings.

Per serving: 510 calories, 20 g protein, 80 g carbohydrates, 12 g fat (1.5 g saturated), 480 mg sodium, 20 g fiber

ROOT FOR YOUR ABS
These matchstick "fries" made of root vegetables pack a wallop of nutrition.

4 LARGE CARROTS, CUT INTO MATCHSTICKS

4 LARGE TURNIPS, CUT INTO MATCHSTICKS

1 TABLESPOON EXTRA-VIRGIN OLIVE OIL SALT AND PEPPER

½ CUP CROUTONS

⅓ CUP GRATED PARMESAN CHEESE

½ TEASPOON GARLIC POWDER

1. Preheat the oven to 425°F. Coat a baking sheet with cooking spray.

2. Mix the carrots, turnips, and oil in a bowl. Season with salt and pepper.

3. Dump the croutons into a resealable plastic bag. Close the bag and crush the croutons with something heavy to transform them into crumbs. Add the Parmesan and garlic powder. Working a handful at a time, add the matchsticks to the bag and shake to coat. Pick the matchsticks out and place on the baking sheet.

4. Bake until tender, 15 to 20 minutes (depending on how thick you cut your vegetables). For crispier fries on all sides, turn the matchsticks halfway through cooking.

Makes 4 servings.

Per serving: 160 calories, 5 g protein, 22 g carbohydrates, 7 g fat (2 g saturated), 340 mg sodium, 6 g fiber

FOOD FACT

Crunchy romaine lettuce delivers eight times the amount of vitamin C found in iceberg lettuce.

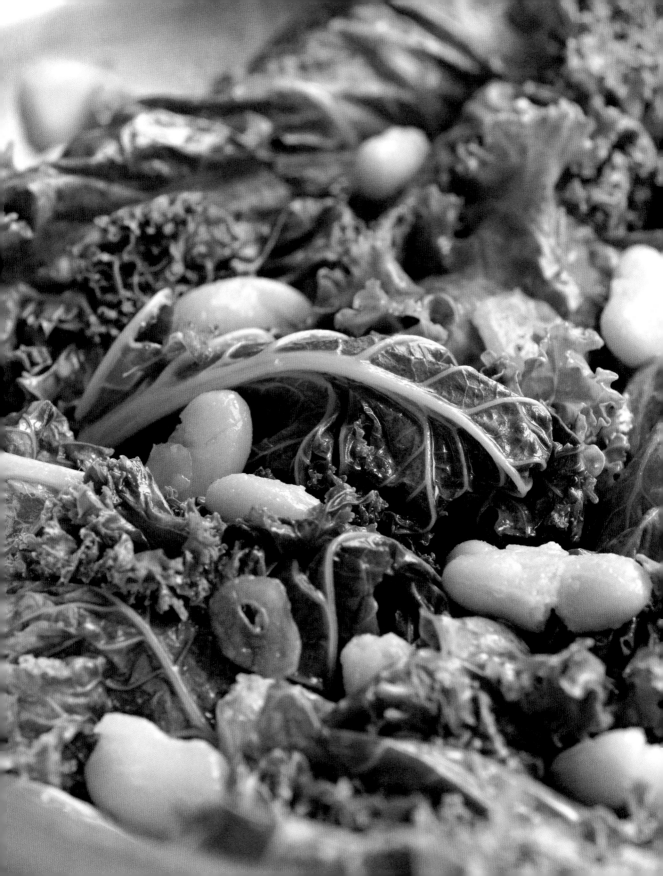

KALE, KALE, THE GANG'S ALL HERE
(Number of Powerfoods: 3)

2 TEASPOONS EXTRA-VIRGIN OLIVE OIL
1 LARGE CLOVE GARLIC, MINCED
1 LARGE BUNCH KALE, CHOPPED
1 CAN (15 OUNCES) NAVY OR CANNELLINI BEANS, RINSED AND DRAINED
SEA SALT AND CRACKED BLACK PEPPER

Heat the oil in a large skillet over medium heat. Add the garlic and cook for 1 minute. Add the kale and sauté until wilted, about 3 to 4 minutes. Add the beans and heat through. Season with salt and pepper. If desired, drizzle a bit more oil over the greens.

Makes 6 servings.

Per serving: 110 calories, 5 g protein, 18 g carbohydrates, 2.5 g fat (0 g saturated), 180 mg sodium, 4 g fiber

IMPROVE YOUR SQUASH GAME

2 POUNDS DELICATA SQUASH
2 POUNDS YUKON GOLD POTATOES
2 TABLESPOONS OLIVE OIL
6 CLOVES GARLIC, SLICED
1 TEASPOON DRIED ROSEMARY
   KOSHER SALT AND GROUND PEPPER

1. Preheat the oven to 425°F. Cut the ends off the squash and cut the squash in half lengthwise. Scoop out the seeds. Cut the squash into 2-inch chunks, leaving the yellowish-green skin on. Cut the potatoes into 2-inch chunks.

2. Dump the squash and potatoes into a roasting pan. Drizzle with the oil. Add the garlic and rosemary; toss to coat.

3. Roast for 20 to 30 minutes or until tender, tossing every 10 minutes to avoid sticking. Season with salt and pepper.

Makes 10 to 12 servings.

Per serving: 120 calories, 3 g protein, 22 g carbohydrates, 2.5 g fat (0 g saturated), 5 mg sodium, 2 g fiber

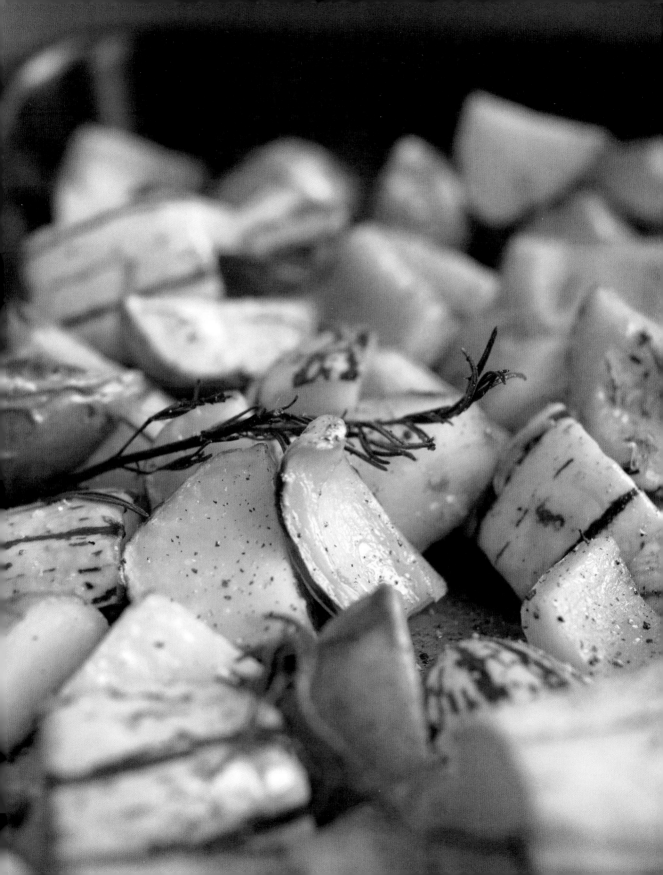

FROM RUSSIA WITH SLAW
(Number of Powerfoods: 2)

- ¼ CUP + 1 TABLESPOON EXTRA-VIRGIN OLIVE OIL
- ¼ CUP BALSAMIC VINEGAR
- 4 TABLESPOONS PREPARED HORSERADISH, DRAINED
- ¼ TEASPOON SEA SALT
- ¼ TEASPOON BLACK PEPPER
- 1 MEDIUM RED ONION, CUT INTO QUARTERS AND SLICED THINLY
- 1 MEDIUM HEAD RED CABBAGE, THINLY SLICED
- 1 LARGE BEET, PEELED AND COARSELY SHREDDED
- ¼ CUP COARSELY CHOPPED PARSLEY

1. Mix ¼ cup oil, vinegar, horseradish, salt, and pepper in a large bowl.

2. Heat the remaining 1 tablespoon oil in a large skillet over medium heat. Cook the onion about 4 minutes or until translucent. Add the cabbage and cook about 6 minutes. It should still be a bit crunchy.

3. Dump the warm cabbage into the bowl with the horseradish mixture. Add the beet and parsley and toss well to combine. Cover with plastic wrap and allow the slaw to marinate at room temperature for an hour before serving.

Makes 8 servings.

Per serving: 130 calories, 2 g protein, 12 g carbohydrates, 9 g fat (1.5 g saturated), 135 mg sodium, 3 g fiber

ABS DIET HALL OF FAME
ROMAINES OF THE DAY
(Number of Powerfoods: 5)

- 2 CUPS CHOPPED ROMAINE LETTUCE HEARTS
- 1 AVOCADO, PITTED, PEELED, AND CHOPPED INTO BITE-SIZE PIECES
- 1 MEDIUM TOMATO, CHOPPED INTO BITE-SIZE PIECES
- ½ CUP CANNED BLACK BEANS, RINSED AND DRAINED
- 2 TABLESPOONS DICED SCALLION
- 1 TABLESPOON CHOPPED CILANTRO
- 1 TABLESPOON EXTRA-VIRGIN OLIVE OIL
- ¼ TEASPOON GRATED LIME ZEST
- 2 TEASPOONS LIME JUICE
- ¼ TEASPOON SALT
- ½ TEASPOON PEPPER

Mix the lettuce, avocado, tomato, beans, scallion, and cilantro in a large bowl. Mix the oil, lime zest and juice, salt, and pepper in a small bowl. Pour over the salad and toss well to coat.

Makes 2 servings.

Per serving: 295 calories, 6 g protein, 24 g carbohydrates, 22 g fat (3 g saturated), 436 mg sodium, 11 g fiber

FOOD FACT

Half of an avocado contains 500 milligrams potassium, 100 more than a banana. Potassium is crucial to reducing high blood pressure, and surveys indicate that Americans fall way short of the recommended 4,700 milligrams per day.

ROSEMARY'S BABY CARROTS

 1 POUND BABY CARROTS
 ¼ CUP BALSAMIC VINEGAR
 1 TABLESPOON EXTRA-VIRGIN OLIVE OIL
 2 TABLESPOONS CRUSHED DRIED ROSEMARY
 2 CLOVES GARLIC, MINCED
 ½ TEASPOON PAPRIKA
    BLACK PEPPER

Preheat the oven to 400°F. Mix everything in a bowl. Spread on a baking sheet and roast for 20 minutes or until tender.

Makes 4 servings.

Per serving: 90 calories, 1 g protein, 15 g carbohydrates, 4 g fat (0 g saturated), 79 mg sodium, 4 g fiber

THE MONSTER MASH

 2 LARGE SWEET POTATOES
 ½ HEAD CAULIFLOWER
 ¾ CUP LOW-SODIUM CHICKEN BROTH
 3 TABLESPOONS FAT-FREE SOUR CREAM
 1 CLOVE GARLIC, MINCED
 ½ TEASPOON GRATED NUTMEG
 1 SCALLION, MINCED
    SALT AND PEPPER

1. Peel and cube the sweet potatoes; cut the cauliflower into florets. Place the cut vegetables in a steaming basket over 1-inch of water in a medium saucepan. Steam for about 10 minutes until tender.

2. Transfer to a large bowl and mash, adding the broth. Stir in the sour cream, garlic, nutmeg, and scallion. Season with salt and pepper.

Makes 4 servings.

Per serving: 122 calories, 4 g protein, 27 g carbohydrates, 0 g fat (0 g saturated), 236 mg sodium, 5 g fiber

How to Mince Garlic

1. After peeling the clove, place it on a cutting board and trim off the tough roots (figure a). **2.** Slice the garlic in thin strips along its length, from root to tip (figure b). **3.** Turn the garlic 90 degrees and cut strips in the other direction. Sprinkle the sticks of garlic with a pinch of salt to keep them from sticking to your knife. **4.** Hold the garlic in place by curling your fingers under and run the knife back and forth over the sticks to mince as finely as you like (figure c).

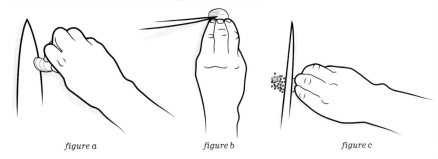

figure a   *figure b*   *figure c*

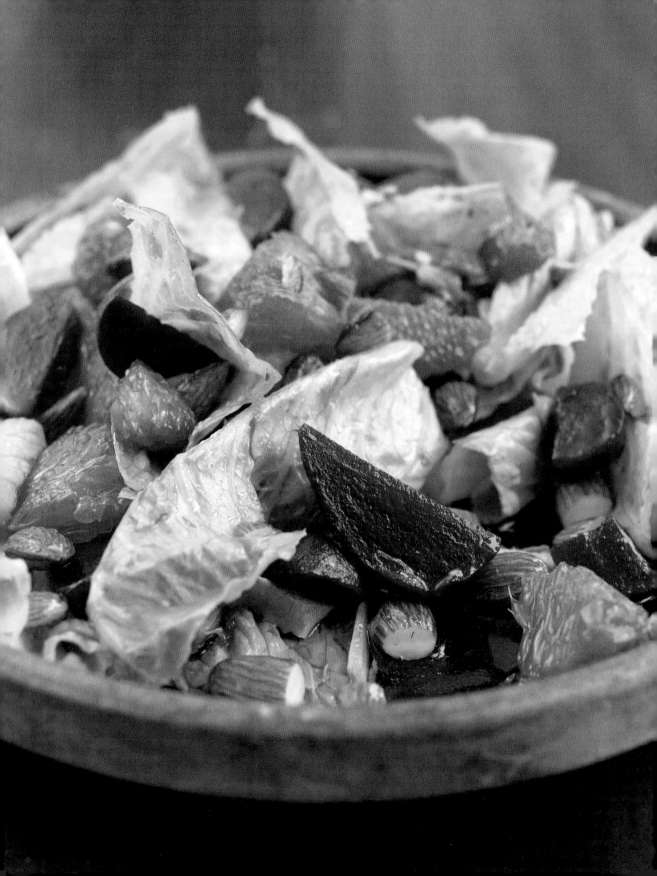

CAN'T BEET THIS SALAD

The juice from the beets and grapefruit makes the dressing.
(Number of Powerfoods: 2)

- **2 CUPS ROMAINE LETTUCE, TORN INTO BITE-SIZE PIECES**
- **¼ CUP JARRED PINK GRAPEFRUIT SALAD OR 1 PINK GRAPEFRUIT, PEELED, SECTIONED, AND DICED**
- **1 CUP CANNED DICED BEETS WITH JUICE**
- **2 TABLESPOONS CHOPPED ALMONDS**

Mix the lettuce, ¼ cup grapefruit with juice, beets with juice, and almonds in a large bowl.

Makes 1 serving.

Per serving: 210 calories, 7 g protein, 33 g carbohydrates, 7 g fat (0.5 g saturated), 310 mg sodium, 9 g fiber

ABS DIET HALL OF FAME CHICKEN SOUP FOR THE BOWL

A perfect weekend meal or one you can use during the week as a premade dinner or heat-up lunch.
(Number of Powerfoods: 3)

1 ROTISSERIE CHICKEN
4 STALKS CELERY, DICED
2 CARROTS, DICED
1 ONION, DICED
2 CLOVES GARLIC, CRUSHED
2 TEASPOONS EXTRA-VIRGIN OLIVE OIL
½ TEASPOON DRIED THYME
½ TEASPOON SALT
½ TEASPOON BLACK PEPPER
⅔ CUP UNCOOKED BROWN RICE
3 CANS (16 OUNCES EACH) LOW-SODIUM CHICKEN BROTH (OPTIONAL)

1. Remove the skin from the chicken. Slice off the breasts, dice, wrap, and refrigerate. Tear apart the rest of the chicken and place pieces of chicken meat in a large pot; cover with water. Bring to a boil, then simmer for 1 hour.

2. Place a colander in a large bowl and strain the chicken liquid into the bowl. Remove the chicken parts, tearing off any meat. Set aside the stock and meat.

3. Wash the pot, then add the celery, carrots, onion, garlic, and oil. Cook over medium-high heat until soft, about 6 minutes.

4. Add the chicken meat (including the refrigerated breast meat), stock, thyme, salt, pepper, and rice. Bring to a boil and then simmer for 30 minutes, adding water or canned broth if needed.

Makes 6 servings.

Per serving: 345 calories, 30 g protein, 25 g carbohydrates, 15 g fat (4 g saturated), 638 mg sodium, 3 g fiber

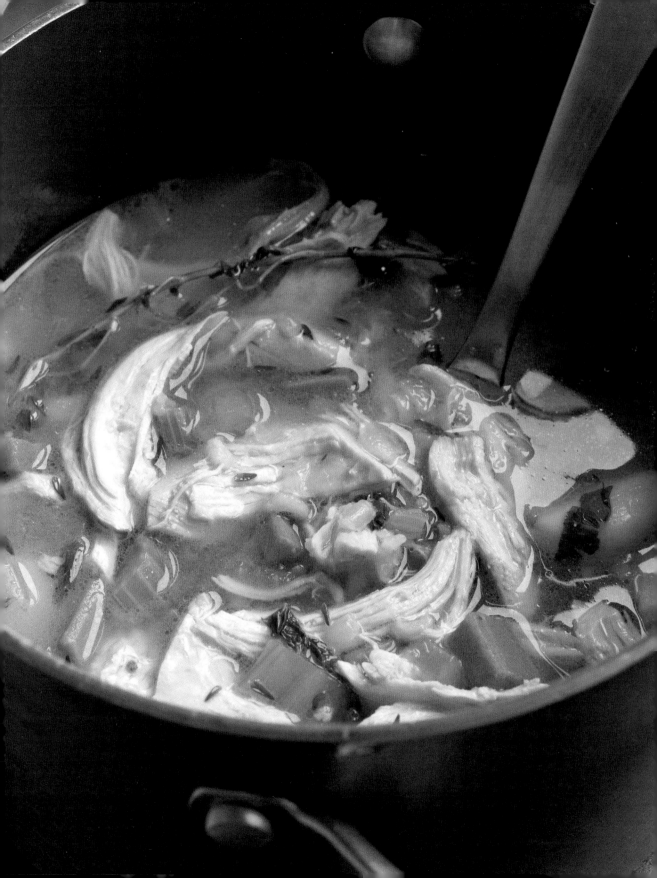

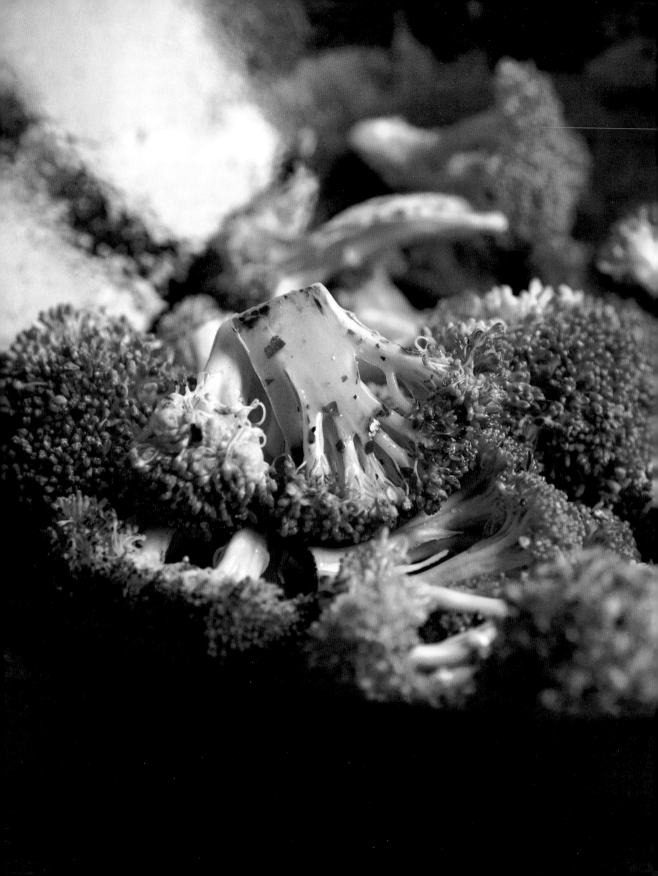

WOK THE BROC
(Number of Powerfoods: 2)

1 LARGE HEAD BROCCOLI
1 TABLESPOON OLIVE OIL
1 TABLESPOON LEMON JUICE
2 DROPS HOT CHILI OIL
1 TEASPOON RED-PEPPER FLAKES
   BLACK PEPPER

1. Cut the broccoli into florets. Peel the stalks and cut into bite-size pieces.

2. Place a steamer basket in a large pot containing 2 inches of water. Bring the water to a boil, then drop in the broccoli and steam for about 1 minute. Drain.

3. Heat the oil in a large nonstick skillet or wok over medium-high heat. Add the broccoli and cook, stirring frequently, for 2 to 3 minutes. Don't overcook. Place in a serving bowl, sprinkle with the lemon juice, and toss with the chili oil and pepper flakes. Season with black pepper.

Makes 4 servings.

Per serving: 70 calories, 3 g protein, 7 g carbohydrates, 4 g fat (1 g saturated), 35 mg sodium, 3 g fiber

FOOD FACT
Kale, broccoli, Brussels sprouts, celery, and peas are rich in a powerful pigment called lutein, which can keep eyes and skin healthy. Research suggests that this nutrient is particularly important for men as they age. After reviewing the diets of 32,000 men, researchers at Johns Hopkins University determined that those who consumed the most lutein-rich vegetables had the lowest risk of developing an enlarged prostate.

IT'S A LENTIL
Serve with crusty bread and a green salad.
(Number of Powerfoods: 3)

1 TABLESPOON OLIVE OIL
1 LARGE CARROT, CHOPPED
1 STALK CELERY, CHOPPED
½ ONION, FINELY CHOPPED
2 CLOVES GARLIC, MINCED
3 CUPS LOW-SODIUM VEGETABLE BROTH
1 CUP DRIED GREEN LENTILS, PICKED OVER AND RINSED
1 CAN (4 OUNCES) GREEN CHILES, DRAINED
SALT AND PEPPER
2 TABLESPOONS RED WINE VINEGAR

1. Heat the oil in a Dutch oven or soup pot over medium heat. Toss in the carrot, celery, onion, and garlic and cook, stirring frequently, for 5 minutes. Add the broth, lentils, and chiles. Season with salt and pepper.

2. Reduce the heat and simmer for 10 minutes. Stir in the vinegar and simmer for 2 minutes.

Makes 4 servings.

Per serving: 221 calories, 11 g protein, 33 g carbohydrates, 5 g fat (0.5 g saturated), 355 mg sodium, 9 g fiber

CALIENTE TORTILLA SOPA
(Number of Powerfoods: 2)

2 CHILE PEPPERS
1½ POUNDS TOMATOES, HALVED
2 TABLESPOONS EXTRA-VIRGIN OLIVE OIL
3 CLOVES GARLIC, SLICED
1 ONION, SLICED
¼ TEASPOON DRIED OREGANO
SALT AND PEPPER
4 CUPS LOW-SODIUM CHICKEN BROTH
2 CUPS COOKED, SHREDDED CHICKEN
2 LIMES
1 CUP BAKED TORTILLA CHIPS
1 CUP CHOPPED CILANTRO
1 AVOCADO, PITTED, PEELED, AND SLICED

1. Place the chiles and tomatoes on a baking sheet and broil until charred on one side. Use metal tongs to turn them over and char the other side.

2. Heat the oil in a Dutch oven or large pot over medium heat. Add the garlic and onion; cook, stirring frequently, for about 7 minutes. Toss in the tomatoes and chiles; use a wooden spoon to crush the charred tomatoes. Season with oregano, salt, and pepper. Add the broth, reduce the heat, and simmer for 25 minutes.

3. Stir in the chicken and cook for another 5 minutes. Squeeze the juice of 1 lime into the broth and season with salt and pepper. Add the tortilla chips and simmer for 1 minute. Serve the soup with lime wedges, cilantro, and slices of avocado.

Makes 6 servings.

Per serving: 409 calories, 23 g protein, 45 g carbohydrates, 12 g fat (2 g saturated), 520 mg sodium, 7 g fiber

FOOD FACT
Foods with bright, rich colors are packed with the most flavonoids and carotenoids, powerful compounds that bind the damaging free radicals in your body, lowering inflammation. (Sorry, Skittles don't count.) Eat nine fistfuls of colorful fruits and vegetables each day and you'll reap the powerful medicinal benefits without having to give up other foods, says Mehmet Oz, MD.

COUSCOUS? YES, YES!
(Number of Powerfoods: 3)

½ CUP COUSCOUS
½ SMALL YELLOW SQUASH, DICED
½ RED BELL PEPPER, DICED
 1 TABLESPOON CRUMBLED FETA CHEESE
 1 TABLESPOON CHOPPED ALMONDS
½ TEASPOON CHOPPED MINT
½ TEASPOON EXTRA-VIRGIN OLIVE OIL
  SALT AND PEPPER

Prepare the couscous according to the package directions. Add the remaining ingredients and toss well to blend.

Makes 2 servings.

Per serving: 210 calories, 8 g protein, 38 g carbohydrates, 3 g fat (1 g saturated), 62 mg sodium, 4 g fiber

QUICK CRANBERRY RELISH

 2 CUPS SWEETENED DRIED CRANBERRIES
½ CUP ORANGE JUICE
¼ CUP WATER
¼ CUP MANDARIN ORANGES, HALVED

Puree the cranberries with the juice and water in a blender, but don't go overboard. You won't be sipping them through a straw. Pour into a bowl and stir in the oranges. Eat immediately or chill for 30 minutes.

Makes 8 servings.

Per serving: 100 calories, 0 g protein, 27 g carbohydrates, 0 g fat (0 g saturated), 0 mg sodium, 2 g fiber

ABS DIET HALL OF FAME
NO-SUFFERIN' SUCCOTASH
(Number of Powerfoods: 3)

 1 CUP FROZEN BABY LIMA BEANS
 1 CUP FROZEN CORN KERNELS
½ SMALL ONION, DICED
 1 CLOVE GARLIC, MINCED
½ RED BELL PEPPER, DICED
 1 TEASPOON EXTRA-VIRGIN OLIVE OIL
½ CUP SHREDDED LOW-FAT
  CHEDDAR CHEESE
  SALT AND PEPPER

1. Place the frozen beans and corn in a colander and run hot water over them until thawed. Drain well.

2. Sauté the onion, garlic, and bell pepper in the oil in a nonstick skillet over medium heat for about 4 minutes. Stir in the vegetables and cheese. Season with salt and pepper.

Makes 2 servings.

Per serving: 256 calories, 14 g protein, 41 g carbohydrates, 5 g fat (1 g saturated), 275 mg sodium, 9 g fiber

ABS DIET POWER TIP
To save fat calories, make your soup a day before eating and chill in the refrigerator. The fat will rise to the top, where it's easy to scrape off with a spoon. To reduce the fat content of creamy soups without losing the creaminess, replace the traditional roux (flour cooked in fat) with pureed soup vegetables.

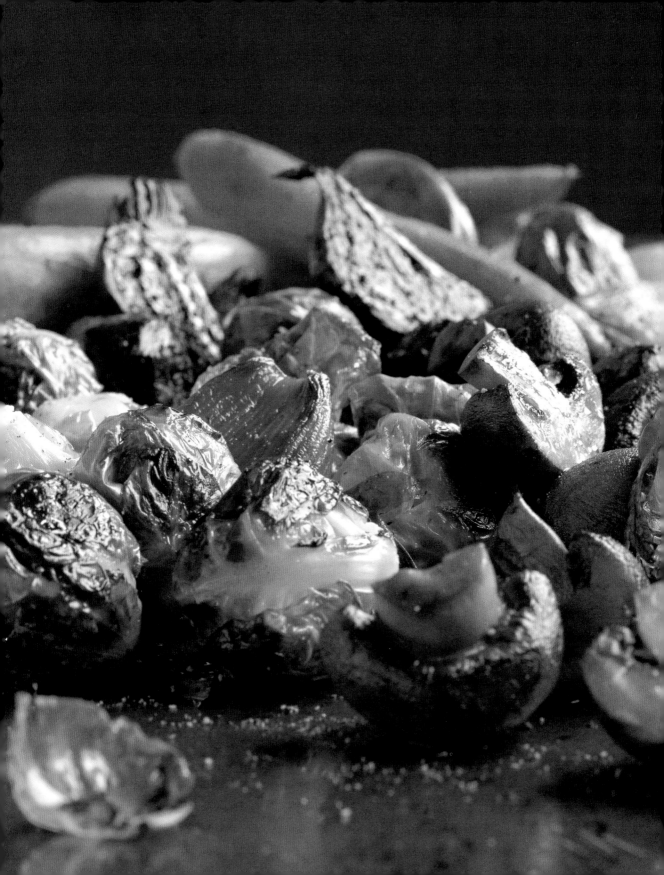

POTLUCK ROAST

Oven-roast almost any vegetables you have on hand—asparagus, broccoli, potatoes, any root vegetable. Use as a main dish with a small side of protein.

1 BUNCH SMALL CARROTS

4 MEDIUM BEETS, TRIMMED
   AND QUARTERED

6 BRUSSELS SPROUTS

8 OUNCES CREMINI MUSHROOMS, HALVED

5 SHALLOTS, HALVED

¼ CUP EXTRA-VIRGIN OLIVE OIL

1 TABLESPOON COARSE SALT
   BLACK PEPPER

Preheat the oven to 400°F.

Spread the vegetables in clusters on a baking sheet. Drizzle with the oil. Sprinkle with salt and pepper.

Roast for about 30 minutes, until the vegetables are tender and caramelized.

Makes 6 servings.

Per serving: 160 calories, 4 g protein, 17 g carbohydrates, 10 g fat (1.5 g saturated), 1,040 mg sodium, 4 g fiber

JIM BEAM BAKED BEANS
(Number of Powerfoods: 3)

- 2 CUPS DRIED NAVY BEANS, PICKED OVER AND RINSED
- 3 STRIPS THICK-CUT BACON, CUT INTO ½-INCH PIECES
- 1 YELLOW ONION, CHOPPED
- 4 CUPS WATER
- 2 BAY LEAVES
- ½ CUP LIGHT MOLASSES
- 1½ TABLESPOONS DRY MUSTARD
- ¼ CUP JIM BEAM BOURBON
- ¾ TEASPOON SALT

1. Put the beans in a large bowl and add cold water to cover by at least 2 inches. Soak overnight. Drain, rinse, and drain again.

2. Cook the bacon in a Dutch oven or large pot over medium heat. When it starts to sizzle, add the onion and cook for 2 minutes, stirring. Add the beans, 4 cups water, and bay leaves. Bring to a boil over high heat. Reduce the heat and simmer for 1 hour and 10 minutes, until the beans have softened. Remove from the heat and discard the bay leaves.

3. Stir in the molasses, mustard, bourbon, and salt. Return the pot to the stove and cook over low heat for 4½ to 5 hours, until very tender.

Makes 12 ⅓-cup servings.

Per serving: 200 calories, 4 g protein, 19 g carbohydrates, 4 g fat (1 g saturated), 197 mg sodium, 6 g fiber

ABS DIET POWER TIP

Add a shot of Tabasco or other hot sauce to soups and stews. Researchers found that levels of insulin—which triggers body fat storage—were lowered by as much as 32 percent following a spicy meal.

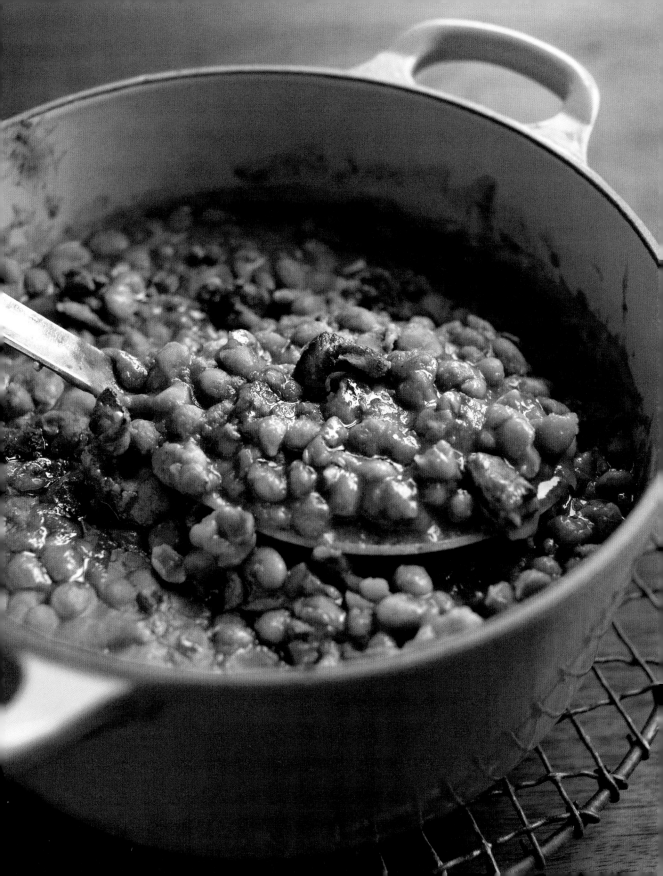

ABS DIET HALL OF FAME
JERRY'S RICE
(Number of Powerfoods: 2)

1 PACKET (14 OUNCES) BOIL-IN-A-BAG
   INSTANT BROWN RICE
   LOW-SODIUM CHICKEN BROTH
1 CUP BROCCOLI FLORETS CUT TO THE
   SIZE OF A THUMB TIP

Follow the package directions for the rice, substituting chicken broth for the recommended amount of water and adding the broccoli after the broth comes to a boil.

Makes 4 servings.

Per serving: 136 calories, 4 g protein, 27 g carbohydrates, 1 g fat (0 g saturated), 80 mg sodium, 2 g fiber

SICILIAN CITRUS SALAD
(Number of Powerfoods: 2)

8 OUNCES PART-SKIM MOZZARELLA
   CHEESE, CUT INTO SMALL CUBES
2 MEDIUM TOMATOES, DICED
2 NAVEL ORANGES, SECTIONED
   AND CHOPPED
2 TABLESPOONS EXTRA-VIRGIN OLIVE OIL
   SEA SALT (OPTIONAL)

Mix the ingredients and season with salt (if using).

Makes 4 servings.

Per serving: 230 calories, 13 g protein, 11 g carbohydrates, 16 g fat (6 g saturated), 55 mg sodium, 2 g fiber

MACHO GAZPACHO
(Number of Powerfoods: 3)

3 LARGE TOMATOES
1 CUP PEELED CHOPPED CUCUMBER
½ CUP REDUCED-FAT PLAIN YOGURT
1 TEASPOON BALSAMIC VINEGAR
1 TEASPOON OLIVE OIL
1 TEASPOON LEMON JUICE
¼ TEASPOON SALT

Seed the tomatoes (cut a crosshatch in the bottom, hold over the sink and squeeze—most of the seeds will come out of the bottom). Core and chop them into rough chunks and chuck them, along with everything else, into the blender. Puree until smooth. Serve cold.

Makes 2 servings.

Per serving: 118 calories, 6 g protein, 17 g carbohydrates, 4 g fat (1 g saturated), 349 mg sodium, 4 g fiber

FOOD FACT
Give watercress a shot for your next salad. A study in the *American Journal of Clinical Nutrition* shows that eating 3 ounces of watercress every day increases levels of the cancer-fighting anti-oxidants lutein and beta-carotene by 100 percent and 33 percent, respectively.

THE TWISTED SISTERS PASTA SALAD

(Number of Powerfoods: 4)

½ POUND SPINACH FUSILLI

2 TABLESPOONS OLIVE OIL

6 CLOVES GARLIC, THINLY SLICED

½ TEASPOON ITALIAN SEASONING

½ 16-OUNCE PACKAGE FROZEN BROCCOLI
AND CAULIFLOWER FLORETS

1 CUP GRAPE TOMATOES, HALVED
SALT AND PEPPER TO TASTE

½ CUP SHAVED PARMESAN CHEESE

1. Cook the pasta according to the package, drain, and reserve some of the pasta water.

2. While the pasta is cooking, warm the olive oil in a large skillet over medium-high heat. Add the garlic and Italian seasoning and stir until the garlic starts to turn brown.

3. Add the broccoli and cauliflower florets. Cook for about 5 minutes, stirring often. Add the grape tomatoes and cook for another 5 minutes, stirring often, until the florets are tender but not mushy. If the vegetables start to stick, add some of the reserved water.

4. Ladle the vegetable mixture over the pasta in a serving plate or bowl. Add salt and pepper to taste. Top with Parmesan cheese.

Makes 4 servings.

Per serving: 330 calories, 14 g protein, 47 g carbohydrates, 11 g fat (9 g saturated), 210 mg sodium, 5 g fiber

BAKED STUFFED SWEET POTATOES

(Number of Powerfoods: 2)

2 LARGE SWEET POTATOES

1 CAN (8 OUNCES) CRUSHED PINEAPPLE

1 TABLESPOON OLIVE OIL

1 TABLESPOON BUTTER

1 TABLESPOON BROWN SUGAR

1 TEASPOON GRATED ORANGE ZEST

½ TEASPOON SALT

2 TABLESPOONS CHOPPED PECANS

1. Preheat the oven to 350°F. Pierce potatoes with a fork.

2. Place the potatoes on a baking dish and bake for 50 minutes or until soft. Remove from the oven and allow to cool enough to handle comfortably.

3. Reduce oven heat to 325°F. Cut the potatoes in half lengthwise. Scoop out the flesh, keeping the skin intact, and place the flesh in a bowl. Add the pineapple, oil, butter, sugar, orange zest, and salt to the potato flesh. Mash with a potato masher, then mix with a spoon or use an electric mixer to combine.

4. Fill the potato skin shells with the mixture so it's overstuffed and coming out the top. Top with the chopped pecans and bake for 15 minutes.

Makes 4 servings.

Per serving: 236 calories, 2 g protein, 38 g carbohydrates, 9 g fat (2 g saturated), 300 mg sodium, 4 g fiber

ABS DIET POWER TIP

Pecans contain some of the highest amounts of disease-fighting antioxidants, according to a USDA study. Add chopped pecans to salads and side dishes, like the Baked Stuffed Sweet Potatoes above.

CHAPTER 8

The New Abs Diet Guide to Healthy Grilling

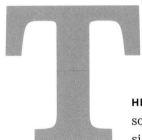

HE IDEA OF GRILLING always sounds great: the open air, the sizzle of flame on flesh, the aroma of smoky meat setting everyone's stomach rumbling. The reality, however, is often less than the fantasy, because many family grill-tenders have only two ways of cooking—raw and burnt.

Well, from here on, burgers as hard as hockey pucks, charred chicken that's still raw inside, and steaks that your rottweiler would have trouble chewing are things of the past. This chapter is designed to introduce you to the many subtleties of grilled food, while quickly and efficiently making you master of the open flame (and, hopefully, giving you enough great tastes and ideas to wean you off that bottle of sugary, calorie-laden commercial barbecue sauce).

Grilling can be a healthful way of cooking because the grates allow much of the saturated fat in meat to drip away. Grilling encourages you and your family to eat more vegetables and fruit because caramelization imparts sweet, smoky flavors that turn mundane vegetables into exotic side dishes. And outdoor cooking delivers social benefits, too: Grilling brings friends and family together. With the tips and innovative recipes in this chapter, you'll be eager to move beyond the basics and develop a mastery of open-flame cooking outdoors that you'll want to share. You'll also discover how you can customize your grillwork

181

for whatever health goal you're looking to achieve, and you'll easily overcome the "I'm too busy to cook" conundrum that keeps so many of us held hostage to the fry-cooks and grease purveyors at America's fast-food restaurants.

But before you spark up your grill, commit these five rules to memory to make cooking easier and more successful:

1. It's all about prep. Once your grill is hot or your guests have arrived, you don't want to be measuring ingredients and you shouldn't be up to your elbows in shrimp marinade and running around your kitchen like a chicken with its head cut off. Doing your prep work well beforehand will make grill cooking much less stressful and the end result far better. So before you light the grill, make sure you have everything you need—the spatulas and tongs at the ready, the little bowls of spices and marinade in place, the veggies cut and rinsed, the meat waiting patiently on a plate under plastic wrap. This is your performance; have your orchestra tuned up.

2. Don't get too hot. If you are using charcoal, avoid cans of charcoal starter or coals presoaked with accelerant—unless you particularly enjoy the flavor of lighter fluid. Instead, invest in a chimney starter. You stuff newspaper in the bottom of this metal cylinder, top that with your briquettes or lump charcoal, and light the newspaper with a match. In 10 minutes, you'll have gray ash coals ready to dump into your grill. If you are using a gas grill, your job is much easier. Light the gas and control the heat with a turn of a knob. With either method, cook with moderate heat to avoid flareups that'll cover your meat with a greasy black film and fail to caramelize it properly.

3. Cook on a clean grate. Using a heavy-duty grill brush, scrub the metal while the grate is warm. Charred food bits on your grill can ruin the taste of meat, fish, and vegetables.

4. Air your meat. Fifteen minutes before grilling, allow the meat to come to near room temperature. Take the meat out of a refrigerator, place it on a plate, and cover with plastic wrap. This will help the meat cook more evenly.

5. Don't poke at it. Use tongs to move your meat around on the grill, not a fork; you'll lose the juices that way and end up with dried, tough meat. And until you've mastered the touch test to gauge doneness on page 203, use a meat thermometer to ensure the meat is cooked to the proper temperature.

Now you're ready to tackle this chapter's delicious grilling recipes, all packed with healthy Abs Diet Powerfoods that deliver flavor and optimal nutrition.

Go ahead: Set something on fire!

Quick Grilling Tip

Here's a quick trick to make any beef, fish, or lamb steak look masterfully prepared: Create the crisscross grill pattern that chefs and cookbook photographers love to show off on their steaks. How to do it: Cook the steak for 2 minutes, then use metal tongs to turn the meat 180 degrees. The thickness of the meat and degree of doneness you prefer will determine length of cooking time. When ready, flip the steak over to cook the other side and repeat the process, turning the steak 180 degrees after 2 minutes of grilling.

Turn the page for 16 New Abs Diet–approved recipes!

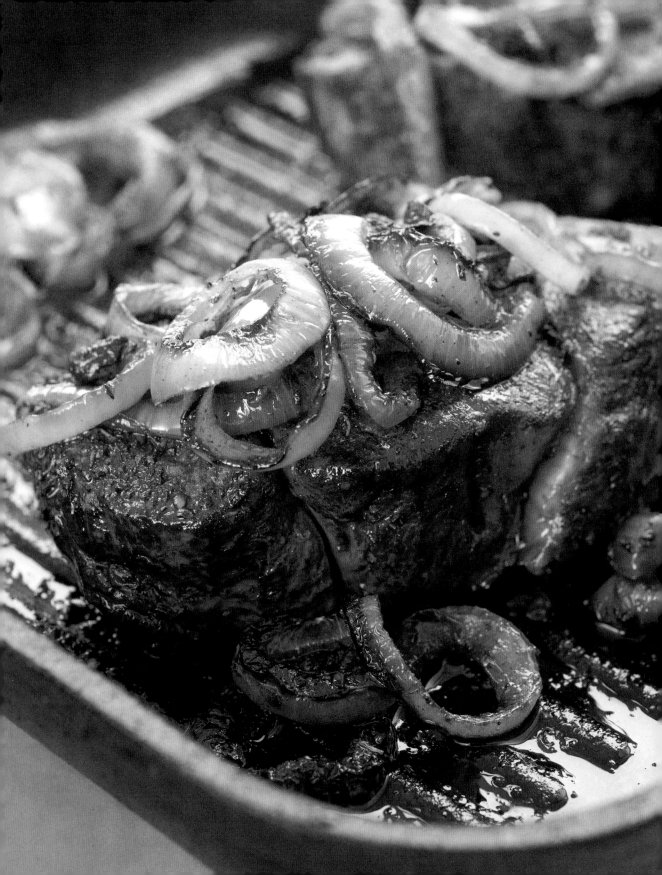

MAKE-MY-DAY FILET WITH GRILLED ONIONS
(Number of Powerfoods: 3)

2 CUPS SLICED VIDALIA ONIONS
  SALT AND PEPPER
1 TEASPOON GARLIC POWDER
½ TEASPOON GROUND CUMIN
½ TEASPOON DRIED OREGANO
¼ TEASPOON CAYENNE
4 PIECES FILET MIGNON
  (4 OUNCES EACH)
1 TEASPOON EXTRA-VIRGIN OLIVE OIL
1 CLOVE GARLIC, THINLY SLICED
1 PACKAGE FRESH SPINACH

1. Coat a grill pan with cooking spray and place over medium heat. Add the onions and season with salt and pepper. Cook, stirring occasionally, until the onions brown. Remove from the heat.

2. Mix the garlic powder, cumin, oregano, cayenne, $1/_8$ teaspoon salt, and $1/_8$ teaspoon pepper in a small bowl. Sprinkle this mixture over each side of the filets.

3. Grill the meat over high heat for about 5 minutes per side or until the desired doneness.

4. Meanwhile, heat the oil and garlic in a large skillet over medium heat. Add the spinach and stir until wilted. Quickly heat up the sautéed onions. Serve the onions on top of the steak and the spinach on the side.

Makes 4 servings.

Per serving: 250 calories, 30 g protein, 14 g carbohydrates, 9 g fat (3 g saturated), 250 mg sodium, 5 g fiber

ABS DIET POWER TIP

To keep meats and vegetables from sticking to your grill, oil it right. Cut an onion in half and stick a long-handled grill fork in the round part. Dip the cut end into a bowl of vegetable oil and rub it over the grates of the grill.

OLD BAY SHRIMP ON THE BARBIE
Serve on a bed of brown rice with steamed sliced yellow squash.
(Number of Powerfoods: 3)

1 CLOVE GARLIC, CRUSHED

1 TABLESPOON OLD BAY SEASONING

2 TABLESPOONS EXTRA-VIRGIN OLIVE OIL

2 TEASPOONS LEMON JUICE

1 POUND LARGE SHRIMP, PEELED AND DEVEINED WITH TAILS LEFT ON

1 LARGE RED BELL PEPPER, CUT INTO 1-INCH PIECES

1 CAN (8 OUNCES) PINEAPPLE CHUNKS, DRAINED

1 LIME, CUT INTO WEDGES

CHOPPED PARSLEY

BROWN RICE (MEDIUM GRAIN)
Per serving: 110 calories, 2 g protein, 23 carbohydrates, 1 g fat (0 g saturated), 0 mg sodium, 2 g fiber

STEAMED YELLOW SQUASH
Per serving: 35 calories, 2 g protein, 8 g carbohydrates, 0.5 g fat (0 g saturated), 0 mg sodium, 3 g fiber

1. Soak 12 bamboo or wooden skewers in water for 30 minutes.

2. Mix the garlic, Old Bay, oil, and lemon juice into a paste in a large bowl. Add the shrimp and toss to coat evenly.

3. Thread the shrimp, bell pepper, and pineapple onto the skewers. Place in a shallow dish, cover, and chill for 30 minutes.

4. Coat a grill with cooking spray before lighting the grill. Place the shrimp skewers on the grill and cook uncovered over medium heat for 3 minutes, turning once.

5. Continue to grill for another 4 minutes or until the shrimp turn pink. Squeeze lime juice over everything and sprinkle with parsley.

Per serving: 220 calories, 25 g protein, 13 g carbohydrates, 8 g fat (1.5 g saturated), 740 mg sodium, 2 g fiber

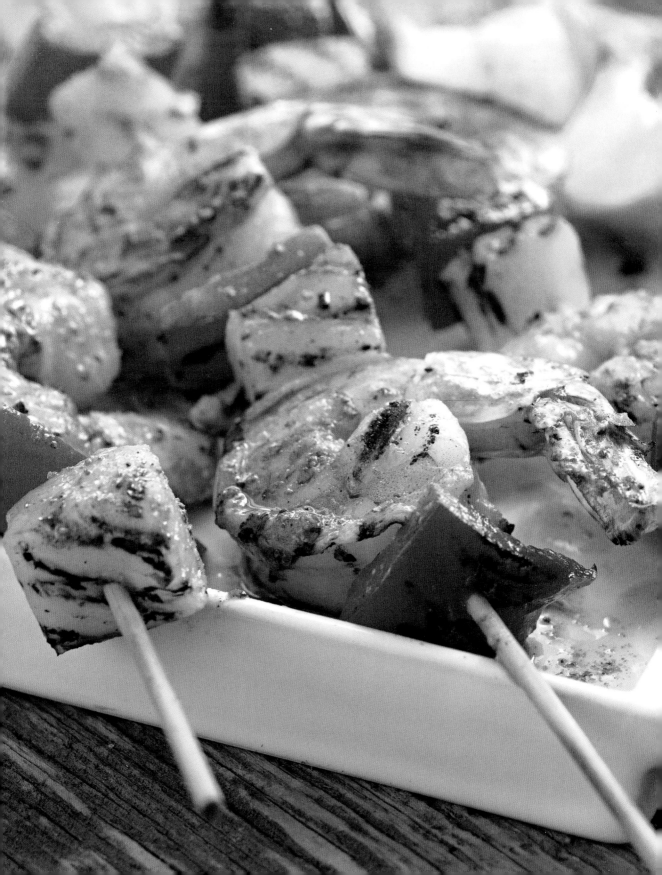

DR. FLANK 'N' STEIN'S MONSTER

It's best to prepare the meat and marinade a day in advance, but in a pinch you can do it a few hours before grill time. Serve the steak with sautéed spinach or kale and Potato Salad with Warm Bacon Dressing, page 197.
(Number of Powerfoods: 3)

2 POUNDS FLANK STEAK

1 TABLESPOON DRIED OREGANO

2 TEASPOONS GROUND CUMIN

1 TEASPOON BLACK PEPPER

1 TABLESPOON SALT

¼ CUP EXTRA-VIRGIN OLIVE OIL

1 TABLESPOON LIGHT BROWN SUGAR

½ CUP WORCESTERSHIRE SAUCE

1 BOTTLE (12 OUNCES) DARK BEER

1. Place the steak on a large cutting board. Score both sides lightly with a sharp knife vertically and horizontally—not too deep but enough to help the marinade absorb into the meat.

2. Sprinkle with a pinch each of the oregano, cumin, pepper, and salt; work the spices into the meat with your fingers.

3. Place the remaining spices in a large resealable bag; add the oil, sugar, Worcestershire sauce, and beer. (If you don't have a plastic bag large enough to hold the meat, use a baking dish and cover it with plastic wrap after adding the marinade.) Place the steak in the bag, seal it, and refrigerate overnight. Turn the bag once or twice during the marinating time.

4. Remove the steak from the bag and discard the marinade. Grill over medium-high heat for 4 minutes per side. Don't overcook. Flank steak should be served medium-rare.

5. Transfer to a platter and let rest for 10 minutes to allow the juices to redistribute. Slice the steak thinly (about ¼-inch slices) across the grain.

Makes 6 servings.

MARINATED STEAK
Per serving: 430 calories, 42 g protein, 9 g carbohydrates, 22 g fat (7 g saturated), 1,270 mg sodium, 1 g fiber

SIDE SPINACH
Per serving: 5 calories, 1 g protein, 1 g carbohydrate, 0 g fat (0 g saturated), 20 mg sodium, 1 g fiber

How to Grill a Healthier Steak

Marinate, say food safety researchers. The American Institute for Cancer Research found that marinating meat briefly before grilling resulted in a 90 percent reduction in cancer-causing compounds known as HCAs (heterocyclic amines). At Kansas State University, scientists marinated steaks in herbs, resulting in 88 percent fewer HCAs, a reduction that directly correlated with the amount of antioxidants in the spiced marinade.

Forgo the store-bought marinades, which are high in sugar and salt, and experiment with your own herb-rich marinade or rub containing some of the herbs in the KSU study: thyme, red and black pepper, allspice, rosemary, chives, paprika, oregano, garlic, and onion.

No time for an overnight marinade? Try this quick method: Mix paprika, cayenne pepper, cumin, dry mustard, salt, pepper, and oregano in a plastic container (experiment with amounts until you find a balance to your liking). When it's time to grill, drizzle olive oil or lemon juice over both sides of your protein and rub in your spice mix. It works for meat and serves as a tasty rub for blackened fish.

YES, YOU CAN GRILL PIZZA
(Number of Powerfoods: 3)

1 POUND WHOLE WHEAT
OR WHITE PIZZA DOUGH
VEGETABLE OIL
EXTRA-VIRGIN OLIVE OIL
1½ CUPS PIZZA SAUCE
2 CUPS SHREDDED PART-SKIM
MOZZARELLA CHEESE

1. Stretch the dough into a rectangular shape (Sicilian pizza style) on a large cutting board. Avoid stretching the dough too thin or you'll risk burning.

2. Dip a wad of paper towels in vegetable oil and carefully oil the grates of a gas grill. Heat the grill on high. Reduce the heat to low-medium, then transfer the stretched pizza dough to the grill, adjusting it carefully with your fingers to retain the rectangular shape. Lightly brush the top of the dough with olive oil, then close the grill top.

3. Cook for 5 to 7 minutes, occasionally lifting the edge of the dough with a metal spatula to check the bottom. You want it brown. The low-medium setting should cook the dough without burning, depending upon the grill.

4. When the bottom of the crust is nice and brown and the top has started to cook, flip the dough over using spatulas and a friend's help. Spread sauce evenly on the dough and top with an even coating of cheese. Close the grill and cook another 5 minutes or until the cheese has melted.

OPTIONAL TOPPINGS:
Chopped chicken; turkey pepperoni; spinach; pineapple and deli ham. Note: If you use vegetables, grill or sauté them separately and add after the pizza has finished cooking. The moisture in vegetables may otherwise make the pizza soggy.

Makes 6 2-slice servings.

Per serving: 350 calories, 16 g protein, 38 g carbohydrates, 16 g fat (5 g saturated), 680 mg sodium, 7 g fiber

THE HEART-HEALTHY BURGER
(Number of Powerfoods: 3)

10 OUNCES AHI TUNA
1 TEASPOON EXTRA-VIRGIN OLIVE OIL
SALT AND PEPPER
2 CIABATTA ROLLS, SLICED
2 TABLESPOONS PREPARED PESTO
2 TABLESPOONS REDUCED-FAT
MAYONNAISE
1 TOMATO, SLICED
¼ RED ONION, THINLY SLICED
2 CUPS MIXED GREENS

1. Divide the tuna into 2 equal portions. Brush with the oil and season with salt and pepper. Grill over high heat for 2 minutes per side. You want the outside of the tuna to be charred crisp and the inside still pink.

2. Toast the rolls and spread the pesto and mayonnaise on them. Slip the tuna, tomato, onion, and greens into the rolls.

Makes 2 servings.

Per serving: 430 calories, 41 g protein, 28 g carbohydrates, 17 g fat, (3.5 g saturated), 540 mg sodium, 4 g fiber

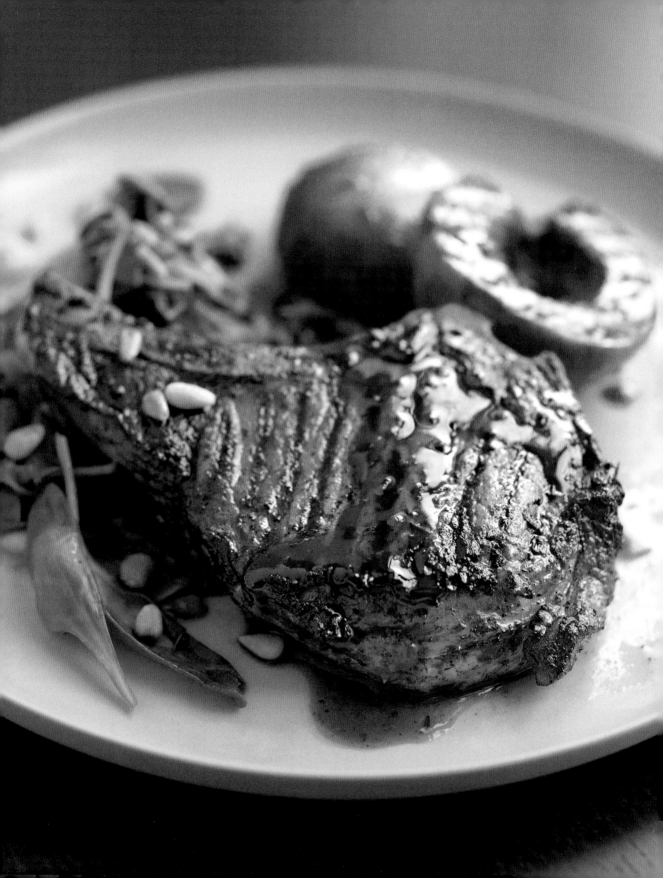

OLD GRAND-DAD'S GLAZED PORK CHOPS AND PEACHES
Serve with steamed spinach topped with toasted pine nuts.
(Number of Powerfoods: 4)

⅓ CUP OLD GRAND-DAD OR OTHER
    BOURBON
¼ CUP HONEY
3 TABLESPOONS LOW-SODIUM
    SOY SAUCE
1 TABLESPOON BROWN SUGAR
1 TABLESPOON EXTRA-VIRGIN OLIVE OIL
½ TEASPOON GROUND GINGER
¼ TEASPOON RED-PEPPER FLAKES
¼ TEASPOON BLACK PEPPER
4 MEDIUM PORK CHOPS ON THE BONE
2 PEACHES, HALVED AND PITTED

1. Mix the bourbon, honey, soy sauce, sugar, oil, ginger, pepper flakes, and black pepper in a large bowl. Transfer about 6 tablespoons of the marinade to a small microwavable bowl. Add pork chops and peaches to the remaining marinade and toss to coat.

2. Grill the pork and peaches over medium-high heat and cook for 5 minutes on each side or until the pork is done.

3. Nuke the remaining marinade on high for 90 seconds and spoon over the pork and peaches.

Makes 4 servings.

PORK CHOPS AND PEACHES
Per serving: 360 calories, 28 g protein, 30 g carbohydrates, 9 g fat (2.5 g saturated), 470 mg sodium, 1 g fiber

SPINACH AND PINE NUTS
Per serving: 40 calories, 5 g protein, 8 g carbohydrates, 1 g fat (0 g saturated), 130 mg sodium, 5 g fiber

WALK-THE-PLANK SALMON WITH GRILLED PINEAPPLE AND ASPARAGUS

See page 203 for grilled pineapple and asparagus recipes.
(Number of Powerfoods: 3)

2 WILD SALMON FILLETS
   (ABOUT 1½ POUNDS)
   SALT AND PEPPER
4 TABLESPOONS GRAINY MUSTARD
6 TABLESPOONS PACKED BROWN SUGAR

GRILLED PINEAPPLE:

1 TABLESPOON EXTRA-VIRGIN OLIVE OIL
¼ TEASPOON GROUND CLOVES
1 TEASPOON GROUND CINNAMON
2 TABLESPOONS HONEY
1 TABLESPOON LIME JUICE
1 RIPE PINEAPPLE
1 TABLESPOON DARK RUM
1 TABLESPOON GRATED LIME ZEST

GRILLED ASPARAGUS:

1 POUND ASPARAGUS,
   TOUGH ENDS TRIMMED
1½ TABLESPOONS EXTRA-VIRGIN OLIVE OIL
   SALT AND PEPPER

FOR THE FISH

1. Soak 1 or 2 cedar planks in cold water for 2 hours. Remove and shake off the water.

2. Rinse the salmon fillets under cold water and pat dry with paper towels. This removes the excess water, which can start to steam the fish.

3. Season the flesh side of the fillets with salt and pepper. Using a brush, spread the mustard over the fish to cover. Make sure to get some on the thick vertical part of the fillet. Crush the brown sugar in a bowl with a fork, then sprinkle over the mustard.

4. Place the cedar planks on a medium-hot grill for 3 minutes, until you can smell smoke. Then turn the planks over and place the coated fillets on the planks skin side down. Cover the grill and cook for about 20 minutes or until the fish is cooked through. (It should reach an internal temperature of 135°F.) If your plank edges start to flame, mist with a spray bottle of water and move to a cooler part of the grill. When done, serve right from the plank.

Makes 4 servings.

Per serving (salmon only): 420 calories, 43 g protein, 20 g carbohydrates, 15 g fat (2 g saturated), 420 mg sodium, 0 g fiber

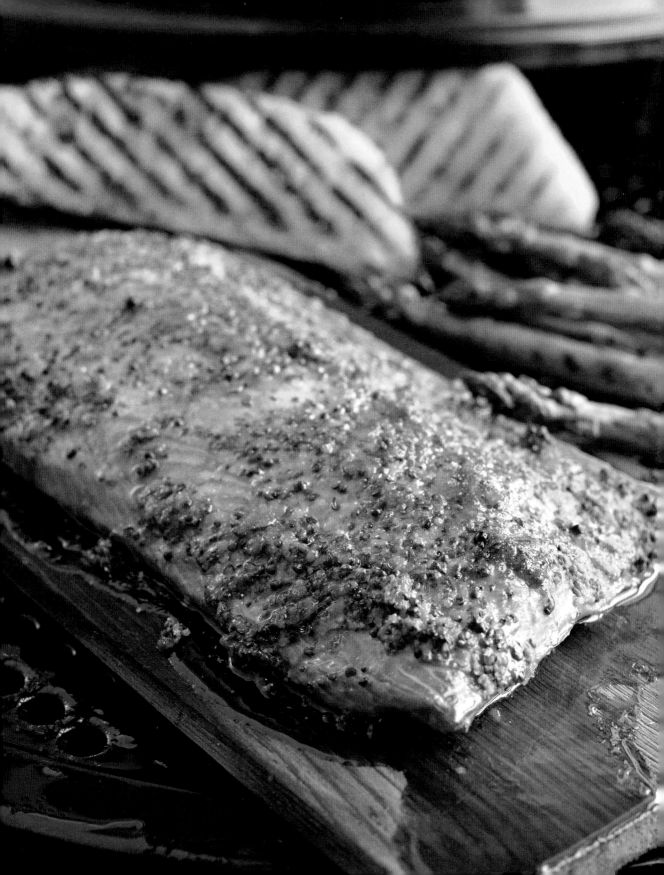

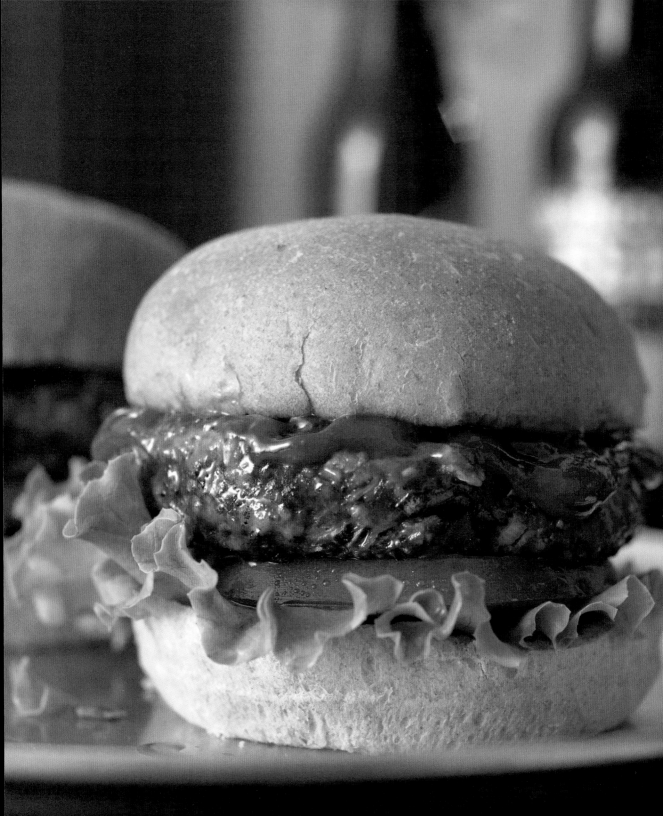

ABS DIET HALL OF FAME **THE OFFICIAL ABS DIET BURGER**

Serve on whole wheat burger buns and top with lettuce and tomato slices.
If you have any extra burgers, wrap them in plastic and freeze for later.
(Number of Powerfoods: 5)

1 EGG
1 POUND LEAN GROUND BEEF
½ CUP ROLLED OATS
⅓ CUP DICED ONION
½ CUP CHOPPED SPINACH
2 TABLESPOONS SHREDDED REDUCED-
FAT MEXICAN-BLEND CHEESE
SALT AND PEPPER

1. Whisk the egg in a large bowl. Add everything else and mix—your hands are the best tools—until well-blended. Form into 4 patties.

2. Place the burgers on a grill over medium-high heat. Cook 4 to 6 minutes per side or to your desired level of doneness.

Makes 4 servings.

Per serving: 263 calories, 27 g protein, 8 g carbohydrates, 13 g fat (5 g saturated), 416 mg sodium, 1 g fiber

ABS DIET POWER TIP

Let the grilled burgers sit for 3 to 4 minutes before eating to allow the juices to redistribute throughout the meat.

LIME-GRILLED TURKEY TACOS WITH AVOCADO SALSA
(Number of Powerfoods: 6)

FOR THE AVOCADO SALSA:

1 AVOCADO, PITTED, PEELED, AND DICED
  JUICE OF 1 LIME
2 TOMATOES, SEEDED AND DICED
½ CUP MINCED SCALLIONS
½ CUP MINCED GREEN BELL PEPPER
½ CUP CHOPPED CILANTRO
  SALT AND PEPPER

FOR THE TURKEY:

½ TEASPOON ONION SALT
½ TEASPOON GARLIC SALT
1 TABLESPOON PAPRIKA
½ TEASPOON CAYENNE
¼ TEASPOON DRIED THYME
¼ TEASPOON BLACK PEPPER
1 POUND TURKEY BREAST TENDERLOINS
1 TABLESPOON EXTRA-VIRGIN OLIVE OIL
1 ONION, SLICED INTO ¼-INCH RINGS
2 JALAPEÑO PEPPERS,
  HALVED LENGTHWISE
2 LIMES, CUT INTO QUARTERS
6 WHOLE WHEAT TORTILLAS OR PITAS
1½ CUPS SHREDDED ROMAINE LETTUCE
½ CUP SOUR CREAM (OPTIONAL)

1. Mix the avocado, lime juice, tomatoes, scallions, bell pepper, and cilantro in a small bowl. Season with salt and pepper. Cover and refrigerate for 30 minutes.

2. Mix the onion salt, garlic salt, paprika, cayenne, thyme, and black pepper. Place the turkey on a plate and drizzle both sides with the oil. Sprinkle with the spice mixture.

3. Place the turkey, onion rings, and jalapeños on the grill over high heat. Grill the turkey for 7 minutes. Squeeze a lime quarter over the meat, turn the pieces, and squeeze another lime quarter over them. Grill for 8 minutes or until a meat thermometer reaches 170°F and the turkey is no longer pink in the center. Grill the onion and jalapeños, turning frequently, until charred. Remove all from the grill.

4. Allow the turkey to rest for 5 minutes, squeeze the remaining lime quarters over the meat, then cut the turkey into ¼-inch strips.

5. Fill the tortillas evenly with turkey, onions, jalapeños, lettuce, avocado salsa, and sour cream (if using).

Makes 6 servings.

Per serving: 280 calories, 24 g protein, 28 g carbohydrates, 12 g fat, (3 g saturated), 460 mg sodium, 6 g fiber

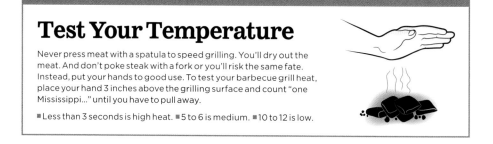

Test Your Temperature

Never press meat with a spatula to speed grilling. You'll dry out the meat. And don't poke steak with a fork or you'll risk the same fate. Instead, put your hands to good use. To test your barbecue grill heat, place your hand 3 inches above the grilling surface and count "one Mississippi…" until you have to pull away.

■ Less than 3 seconds is high heat. ■ 5 to 6 is medium. ■ 10 to 12 is low.

POTATO SALAD WITH WARM BACON DRESSING

for Dr. Flank 'N' Stein's Monster, page 188

2 POUNDS RED POTATOES, CUT INTO LARGE CHUNKS

2 STRIPS BACON, CHOPPED

1 SMALL RED ONION, CHOPPED

1 CLOVE GARLIC, CHOPPED

3 TABLESPOONS CIDER VINEGAR

3 TABLESPOONS APPLE JUICE

1 TABLESPOON STONE-GROUND MUSTARD

¼ CUP CHOPPED PARSLEY

⅛ TEASPOON SALT

1. Set a vegetable steamer in a medium saucepan. Fill with water to just below the steamer. Place the potatoes on the steamer. Cover and bring to a boil over high heat. Reduce the heat to medium-high. Cook for 15 to 20 minutes, or until tender. Transfer to a large bowl and allow to cool for 10 minutes.

2. Meanwhile, in a medium nonstick skillet set over medium heat, cook the bacon for 3 minutes. Add the onion and garlic. Cook, stirring, for 3 minutes, or until the onion is soft and the bacon is crisp. Reduce the heat to low. Add the vinegar, apple juice, mustard, parsley, and salt. Cook for 2 minutes, or until heated through. Pour over the potatoes. Toss to evenly coat.

Makes 6 servings.

Per serving: 129 calories, 4 g protein, 27 g carbohydrates, 1 g fat (0.5 g saturated), 141 mg sodium, 3 g fiber

HOLY MACKEREL, THAT'S GOOD!

Serve with brown rice and steamed broccoli to elevate this meal to 4 Powerfoods.

½ TEASPOON GRATED LEMON ZEST

1½ TABLESPOONS LEMON JUICE

⅓ CUP + 2 TABLESPOONS EXTRA-VIRGIN OLIVE OIL

2 TABLESPOONS CHOPPED THYME LEAVES

SALT AND PEPPER

4 WHOLE MACKEREL (ABOUT 1 POUND EACH)

3 LEMONS SLICED INTO 24 THIN SLICES

1. Mix the lemon zest and juice in a small bowl. Whisk in ⅓ cup oil. Add thyme and season with salt and pepper.

2. Use a sharp knife to cut shallow diagonal slits spaced 2 inches apart into both sides of each fish. Brush the fish with 2 tablespoons oil and sprinkle with salt and pepper. Sprinkle the cavities with salt and pepper and place 2 thin lemon slices in each. Place 2 lemon slices on each side of each fish and hold in place using kitchen string.

3. Grill over medium-high heat for about 5 minutes per side or until the fish is cooked through. Move the fish to a large platter, snip off the string if it hasn't burned off, and drizzle with the lemon vinaigrette.

Makes 8 servings.

Per serving (fish only): 580 calories, 42 g protein, 2 g carbohydrates, 44 g fat, (9 g saturated), 240 mg sodium, 1 g fiber

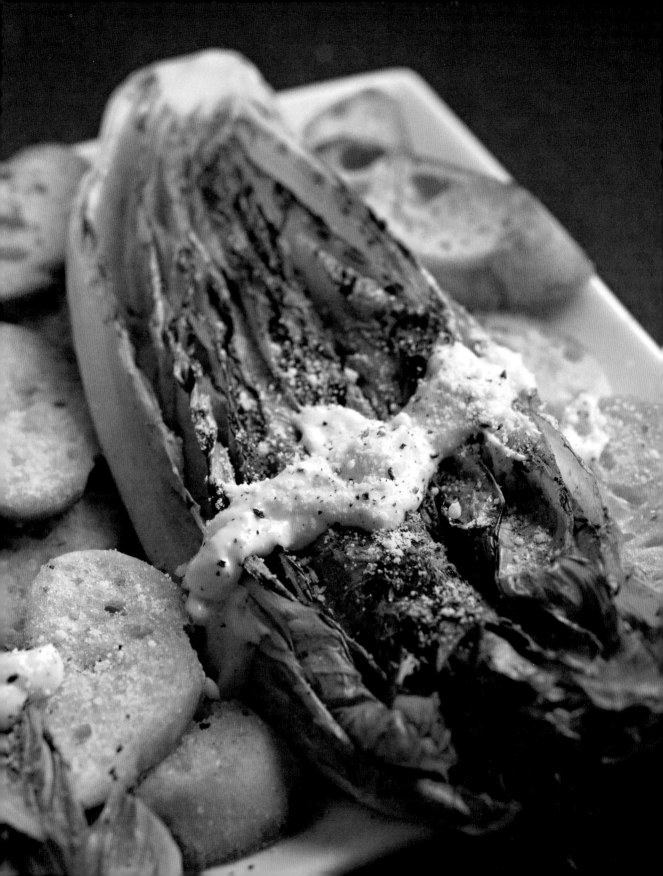

YES, YOU CAN GRILL CAESAR SALAD

Goes great with steak and grilled seafood. To make the salad a meal,
add grilled chicken breast cut into bite-size chunks.
(Number of Powerfoods: 3)

1 FRENCH BAGUETTE
2 TABLESPOONS EXTRA-VIRGIN OLIVE OIL
1/3 CUP LIGHT MAYONNAISE
1/3 CUP GRATED PARMESAN CHEESE
3 TABLESPOONS LEMON JUICE
1 TEASPOON ANCHOVY PASTE
1/4 TEASPOON BLACK PEPPER
1 CLOVE GARLIC, HALVED
1 PACKAGE ROMAINE LETTUCE HEARTS

1. Cut the bread into $1/2$-inch slices. Brush both sides of the slices lightly with the oil. Grill over medium heat for 3 minutes per side to toast. Set aside to cool.

2. Mix the mayonnaise, cheese, lemon juice, anchovy paste, pepper, and any remaining oil in a large bowl until smooth; refrigerate until needed.

3. Rub the cut garlic over both sides of each bread slice. Cut the bread into $1/2$-inch cubes.

4. Cut each head of the romaine lettuce in half lengthwise. Grill about 5 minutes or until wilted and slightly browned on each side, turning once. Place each half on a salad plate, drizzle with the dressing, and toss on the croutons. Finish with a sprinkle of cheese.

Makes 4 servings.

Per serving: 245 calories, 7 g protein, 20 g carbohydrates, 14 g fat (3 g saturated), 420 mg sodium, 3 g fiber

LEMONY LAMB LOLLIPOPS
(Number of Powerfoods: 3)

1 CUP LOW-FAT PLAIN YOGURT
1 TABLESPOON LEMON JUICE
⅛ TEASPOON SWEET OR HOT PAPRIKA
⅛ TEASPOON GROUND CUMIN
8 RIB LAMB CHOPS
1½ TEASPOONS SALT
½ TEASPOON BLACK PEPPER
  MINT SPRIGS (OPTIONAL)

1. Mix the yogurt, lemon juice, paprika, and cumin in a bowl and refrigerate until needed.

2. Sprinkle both sides of the lamb chops with salt and pepper. Grill over medium heat for 5 minutes per side or until cooked through. Serve with the yogurt sauce.

Makes 4 servings.

Per serving: 450 calories, 27 g protein, 5 g carbohydrates, 35 g fat (18 g saturated), 850 mg sodium, 0 g fiber

ABS DIET POWER TIP

A meal-ruining inferno can happen when fat drippings meet hot coals. To minimize flare-ups, trim visible fat before grilling. When flame-ups occur, move the meat to another part of the grill or to a warming rack until the fat burns off the grill. Don't try to douse the flame; water and hot grease don't mix.

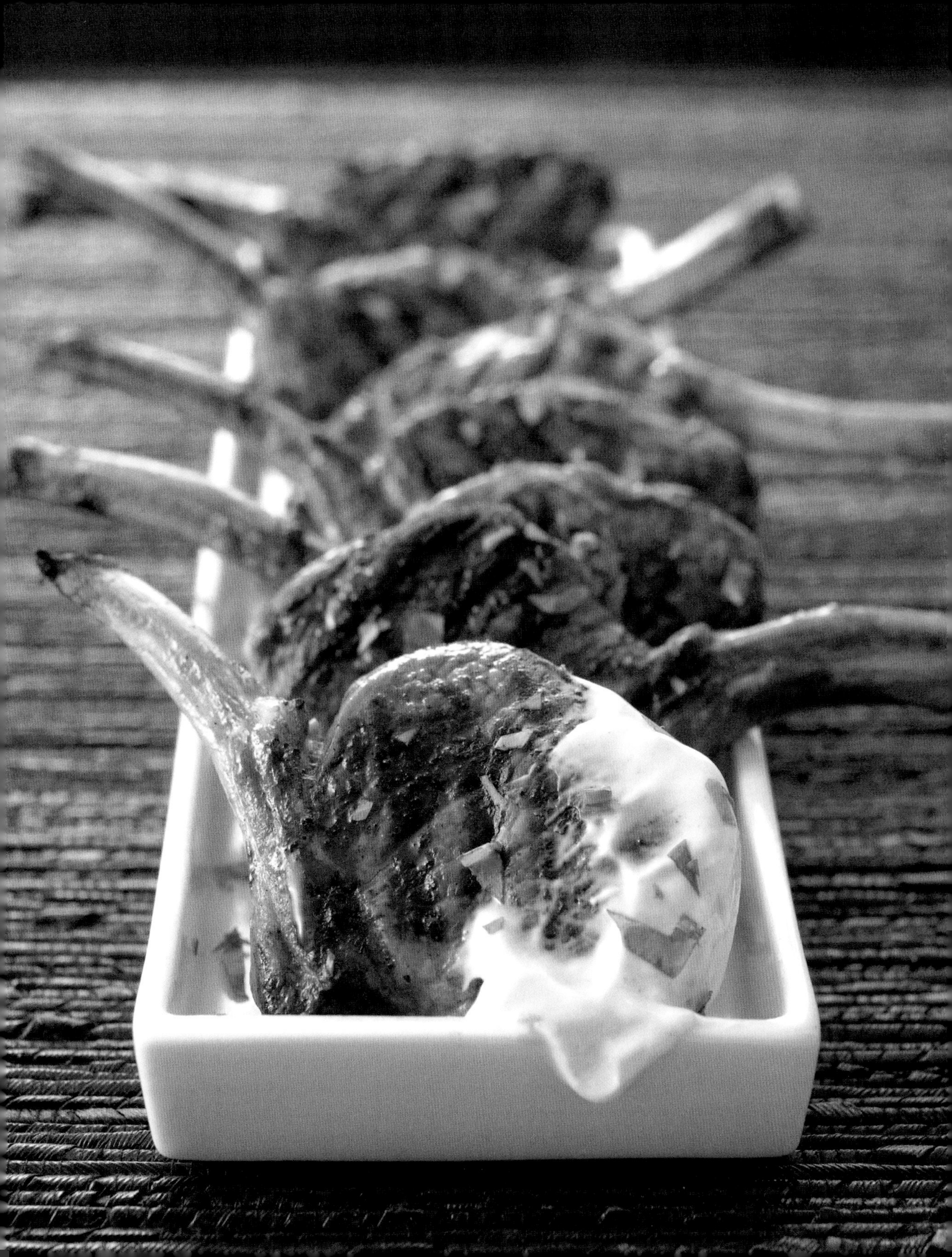

THE WEIGHT-LOSS BURGER

Stoke your metabolic engine with this high-protein meal and cut the carbs by going bun-free.
(Number of Powerfoods: 4)

10 OUNCES GROUND BUFFALO
 1 TEASPOON EXTRA-VIRGIN OLIVE OIL
   SALT AND PEPPER
 2 SLICES RED ONION
 2 EGGS
 4 LARGE ROMAINE LETTUCE LEAVES,
   RIBS REMOVED
⅓ CUP SHREDDED SHARP
   CHEDDAR CHEESE
   KETCHUP
   DIJON MUSTARD

1. Form the meat into 2 patties. For medium-rare burgers, allow the meat to rest at room temperature for about 30 minutes. Brush with the oil and season with salt and pepper.

2. Grill over high heat for 4 minutes per side. At the same time, grill the onion slices until lightly charred.

3. Fry the eggs in a nonstick skillet until the desired degree of doneness.

4. For each serving, overlap 2 lettuce leaves on a plate, top with the burger, fried egg, cheese, onion, ketchup, and mustard. Fold the lettuce over the burger and eat with both hands.

Makes 2 servings.

Per serving: 390 calories, 42 g protein, 7 g carbohydrates, 21 g fat (8 g saturated), 450 mg sodium, 1 g fiber

THE RECOVERY BURGER

The carb-protein balance makes this a perfect postworkout meal. For even cooking, allow the patties to rest at room temperature for about 30 minutes before grilling.
(Number of Powerfoods: 3)

10 OUNCES LEAN GROUND TURKEY
 4 TABLESPOONS TERIYAKI SAUCE
 2 SLICES FRESH PINEAPPLE
 2 THICK SLICES RED ONION
 2 WHOLE WHEAT BUNS, TOASTED
½ JALAPEÑO PEPPER, THINLY SLICED
 2 SLICES SWISS CHEESE

1. Form the ground turkey into 2 patties. Grill over high heat for 4 minutes per side, basting frequently with 2 tablespoons teriyaki sauce. At the same time, grill the pineapple and onion slices until lightly charred.

2. Put each burger on a bun and layer on the onion, pineapple, jalapeño, and cheese. Top with the remaining 2 tablespoons teriyaki sauce.

Makes 2 servings.

Per serving: 510 calories, 39 g protein, 40 g carbohydrates, 22 g fat (9 g saturated), 1,770 mg sodium, 5 g fiber

ABS DIET POWER TIP

Marinate food for at least 30 minutes before cooking. If you are using a rub on meat, apply it immediately before you toss the meat on the grill. The salt in the rub will draw moisture out of the meat if left on the food too long before cooking, making it dry.

GRILLED PINEAPPLE AND ASPARAGUS

For ingredient list, see Walk-the-Plank Salmon, page 192.

FOR THE PINEAPPLE

1. Mix the oil, cloves, cinnamon, honey, and lime juice in a large bowl.

2. Cut off the leaves and base of the pineapple. Stand the fruit upright and cut off the skin using a large sharp knife. Be sure to cut off the hard pineapple "eyes." Then cut the fruit in half lengthwise. Place each half cut side down and cut into four wedges lengthwise. Place all 8 wedges in the bowl of marinade and stir to coat.

3. Grill the wedges over high heat until golden brown, brushing often with marinade and turning the pieces several times, about 10 minutes total.

4. Place on a platter, brush with the rum, and sprinkle with the lime zest.

Makes 8 servings.

Per serving: 90 calories, 1 g protein, 20 g carbohydrates, 2 g fat (0 g saturated), 0 mg sodium, 2 g fiber

FOR THE ASPARAGUS

Brush the asparagus with oil and season with salt and pepper. Grill over high heat for 3 to 4 minutes, turning once or twice, until tender and slightly charred.

Makes 4 servings.

Per serving: 70 calories, 2 g protein, 4 g carbohydrates, 5 g fat (0.5 g saturated), 0 mg sodium, 2 g fiber

A Handy Meat Thermometer
To check "doneness," poke the meat and then your hand

Too rare: Poke the soft area between your thumb and index finger when your hand is relaxed.

Medium rare: Stretch your fingers halfway open and poke the same place for a firmer but still squishy feel.

Medium: Spread your hand all the way open and poke.

Well done: Make a fist and poke.

CHAPTER 9

The New Abs Diet Dinners and Desserts

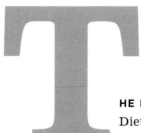

HE BEAUTY OF THE NEW ABS Diet is its simplicity. Unlike most diet plans that declare "don't eat this, don't eat that," the Abs Diet tells you exactly what to eat in order to lose weight and improve your health. It's this positive approach to healthy eating that makes incorporating the diet's principles into your life extremely easy and intuitive. That comes in especially handy when dinnertime rolls around. Dinner, after all, is the most complicated of the three squares: It's the meal during which we catch up on our days and launch our nights, and it ought to look, feel, and taste substantial. Sure, you can have omelets and toast ("breakfast for dinner") or soup and salad ("lunch for dinner"), but sometimes you want a real dinner for dinner. And for good reason.

The evening meal should be a celebration of sorts. After all, you've worked hard all day long dealing with craziness and pressure. There's nothing wrong with rewarding yourself for making it through another grueling day and taking some time out to enjoy food with your friends and family. Thing is, when most of us bust our butts on the job, it's not the way our granddads busted theirs back in the day—using their muscles to swing hammers and pickaxes or toil in the steel mills and dockyards. They burned a ton of calories bringing home the bacon. Their bodies could handle a big meal—even one with a lot of greasy bacon—without turning flabby. Things have changed dramatically.

It's not the same for most of us who toil at a desk for 8 hours or more flexing our finger muscles over a computer keyboard. We are just not doing the heavy manual labor that once helped us burn through so many calories. What's more, we have access to so much more food and more kinds of food than Americans did 50 or more years ago. In 1957, for example, the typical hamburger was 1 ounce of cooked ground beef; today, it weighs 6 ounces. Today, the typical American consumes 45 more pounds of added sugars than he did in the 1950s. So how do we enjoy the kind of meal we rightly deserve without consuming loads of calories we don't need?

That's where this chapter can make life easy. Each of the recipes here is based on the 12 Abs Diet Powerfoods; each is packed with fat-burning, muscle-building, hunger-satisfying nutrients. Each of the recipes in this chapter in particular looks deliciously impressive—as though you've spent years training in Hell's Kitchen. And the majority of them take your busy life into consideration: They can be whipped up in no time at all.

Now, a caveat: Just because you can cook up dinner in no time doesn't mean you should wolf down dinner in no time. One of the best ways to bust calories from your diet is to slow down while you're eating. A study at the University of Rhode Island found that consciously slowing down between bites decreases a person's calorie intake by 10 percent. And a University of Massachusetts study found that when you eat while watching TV, you scarf down an average of 288 more calories. (Just watching *American Idol* twice a week at dinner can cost you 2 pounds over the course of a single season—or approximately the same weight by volume as Ryan Seacrest's hair gel.)

And while these easy-to-make, nutrition-packed, fat-busting dinners are all delicious, if you're following the Abs Diet principles—fueling up throughout the day with six smart, strategic meals and snacks—you won't be ravenous the second you walk through the door and you won't be tempted to pig out at dinnertime. That's important, because after dinner, you've got a job to do.

You've got to save room for dessert!

Quick Dinner Tip

Add lean protein to pasta to reduce the high-glycemic load of noodles. When researchers in Britain added tuna to a pasta dish, they found that the meal's glycemic index was cut in half. The protein in the tuna slows the absorption of sugar into the bloodstream, moderating the typical blood sugar spike that can signal the body to store fat.

Turn the page for 35 New Abs Diet–approved recipes!

ABS DIET HALL OF FAME **THREE AMIGOS CHILI**
(Number of Powerfoods: 5)

1 TABLESPOON EXTRA-VIRGIN OLIVE OIL

1 SMALL ONION, DICED

1 POUND GROUND TURKEY BREAST

1 CAN (14.5 OUNCES) DICED TOMATOES WITH JALAPEÑOS

1 CAN (10.5 OUNCES) CHICKPEAS, RINSED AND DRAINED

1 CAN (10.5 OUNCES) BLACK BEANS, RINSED AND DRAINED

1 CAN (10.5 OUNCES) KIDNEY BEANS, RINSED AND DRAINED

1 CAN (14 OUNCES) LOW-SODIUM CHICKEN BROTH

½ TEASPOON SALT

½ TEASPOON GROUND CUMIN

⅛ TEASPOON GROUND CINNAMON

HOT SAUCE

Heat the oil in a large saucepan over medium-low heat. Add the onion and cook until soft, about 3 to 5 minutes. Add the turkey and cook, breaking up the pieces with a wooden spoon, until browned, about 5 minutes. Add the tomatoes with juice, beans, broth, and spices. Stir and bring to a boil, then reduce the heat and simmer for 20 minutes. Serve with hot sauce.

Makes 6 servings.

Per serving: 293 calories, 31 g protein, 32 g carbohydrates, 5 g fat (0 g saturated), 788 mg sodium, 11 g fiber

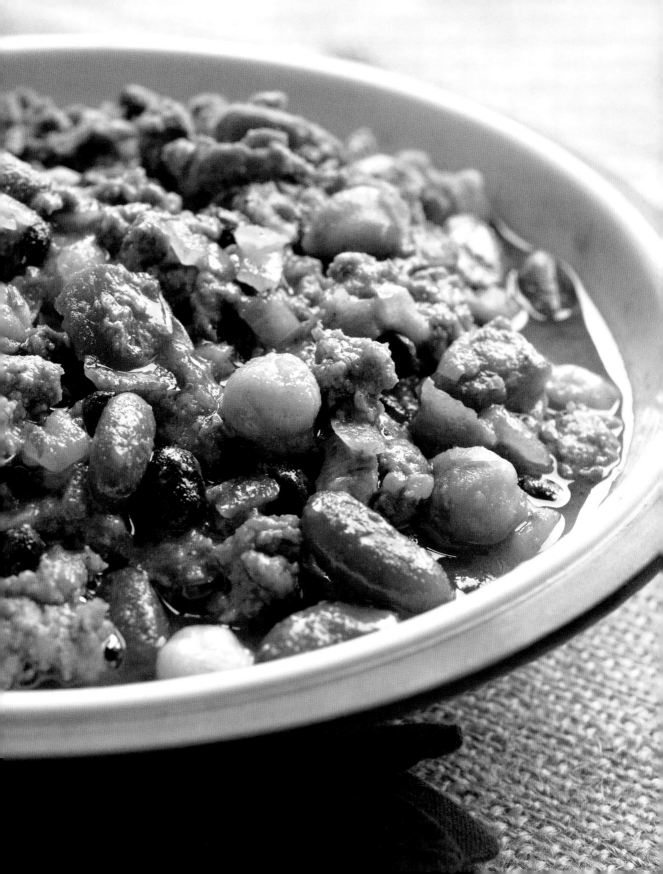

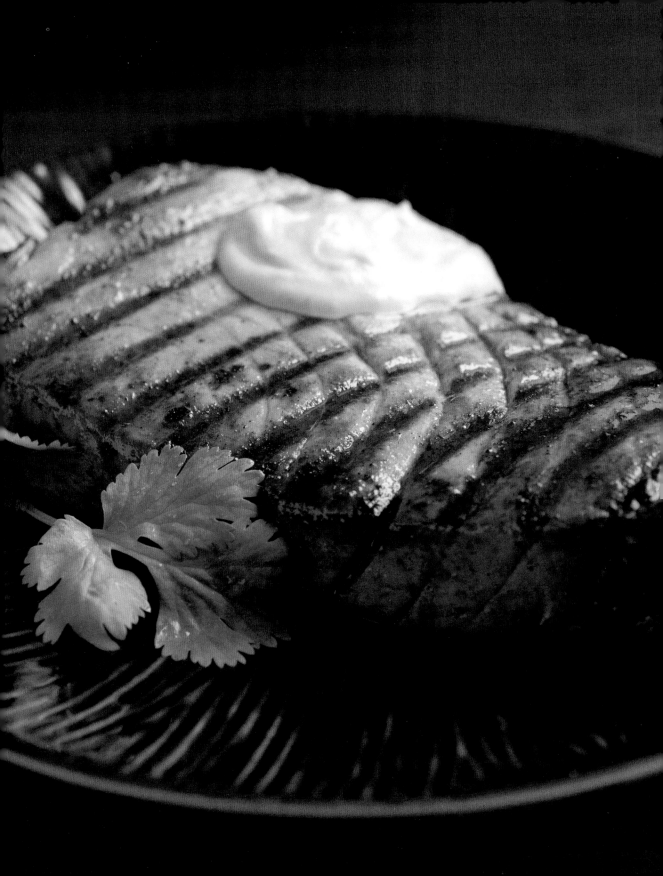

TUNA WITH WASABI

The more wasabi you use, the clearer your sinuses will feel.
(Number of Powerfoods: 2)

- 2 TABLESPOONS REDUCED-SODIUM SOY SAUCE
- 2 TABLESPOONS RICE VINEGAR
- 1 TABLESPOON SUGAR
- ½ TEASPOON TOASTED SESAME OIL
- ½ TEASPOON GROUND GINGER
- 1½ POUNDS TUNA STEAKS
- ¼ CUP REDUCED-FAT SOUR CREAM
- ½ TEASPOON WASABI PASTE

1. Mix the soy sauce, vinegar, sugar, oil, and ginger in a glass baking dish. Add the tuna steaks, turning to coat. Cover and allow to marinate in the refrigerator for 30 minutes, turning twice. Mix the sour cream and wasabi in a small bowl.

2. Coat a grill pan with cooking spray. Remove the tuna from the dish and discard the marinade. Place the steaks on the hot grill pan. Cook for 6 minutes, turning once, for medium-rare. Serve with the wasabi sauce.

Makes 6 servings.

Per serving: 194 calories, 27 g protein, 4 g carbohydrates, 7 g fat (2 g saturated), 227 mg sodium, 0 g fiber

SON-OF-A-GUN STEW (JAMBALAYA)
(Number of Powerfoods: 2)

½ POUND ANDOUILLE-STYLE
   SPICY CHICKEN SAUSAGE

1 PACKAGE (16 OUNCES) FROZEN PEPPER
   STIR-FRY MIX (YELLOW, GREEN,
   AND RED BELL PEPPERS WITH ONION)

2 STALKS CELERY, CHOPPED

1 CAN (14.5 OUNCES) DICED TOMATOES
   WITH JALAPEÑOS

1 POUND BONELESS, SKINLESS CHICKEN
   BREASTS, CUT INTO 1-INCH CUBES

2 CUPS WATER

1 PACKAGE (8 OUNCES) ZATARAIN'S NEW
   ORLEANS STYLE JAMBALAYA RICE MIX

1 POUND FROZEN PEELED AND
   COOKED SHRIMP, THAWED

1. Halve the sausage lengthwise and cut into ½-inch slices. Place in a large slow cooker and stir in the peppers, celery, tomatoes with juice, chicken, water, and the spice packet from the rice mix. Cover and cook on low for 6 hours.

2. Stir in the rest of the rice mix, cover, and cook on high for 35 minutes. Stir in the shrimp and cook for 5 minutes.

Makes 6 servings.

Per serving: 360 calories, 42 g protein, 36 g carbohydrates, 4.5 g fat (1.5 g saturated), 1,190 mg sodium, 3 g fiber

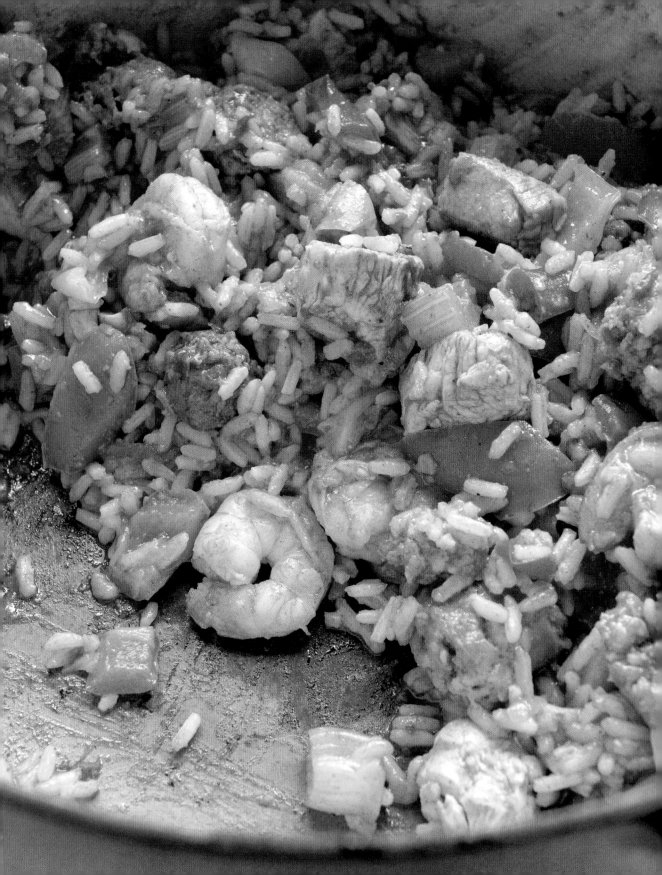

GREEN GOBBLER LASAGNA
(Number of Powerfoods: 5)

1 EGG
1½ CUPS FAT-FREE RICOTTA CHEESE
½ TEASPOON GROUND BLACK PEPPER
1 TABLESPOON MINCED GARLIC
1 TABLESPOON DRIED OREGANO
1 CAN (28 OUNCES) CRUSHED TOMATOES
6 OVEN-READY LASAGNA NOODLES
3 CUPS TORN BABY SPINACH LEAVES
1½ CUPS FINELY CHOPPED
   SKINLESS ROAST TURKEY
¾ CUP SHREDDED PART-SKIM
   MOZZARELLA CHEESE

1. Preheat the oven to 375°F. Coat a 12-by-8-inch baking dish with cooking spray.

2. In a small bowl, beat the egg, then mix with the ricotta and pepper until well-blended. Stir in the garlic and oregano.

3. Spread ¼ cup of tomatoes over the bottom of the baking dish and place three noodles overlapping slightly on top. Spread on half of the ricotta mixture, half of the spinach, half of the turkey, half of the remaining tomatoes, and half of the cheese. Top with the remaining noodles, ricotta mix, spinach, turkey, tomatoes, and cheese.

4. Loosely cover the dish with aluminum foil and bake for 45 minutes. Let sit for 5 minutes before serving.

Makes 6 servings.

Per serving: 276 calories, 28 g protein, 26 g carbohydrates, 6.8 g fat (3.4 g saturated), 619 mg sodium, 4 g fiber

PENNE AND THE JETS
(Number of Powerfoods: 6)

12 OUNCES WHOLE WHEAT PENNE PASTA
2 TABLESPOONS EXTRA-VIRGIN OLIVE OIL
1 CLOVE GARLIC, MINCED
½ CUP SUN-DRIED TOMATOES, CHOPPED,
   SOAKED IN WATER, AND DRAINED
2 TABLESPOONS CHOPPED FRESH PARSLEY
1 TABLESPOON CHOPPED FRESH BASIL
10 OUNCES BABY SPINACH
4 OUNCES FETA CHEESE, CRUMBLED
½ CUP KALAMATA OLIVES, PITTED
½ CUP CHICKPEAS

Cook the penne per package directions. Drain. Heat the oil in a large skillet over medium-high heat. Sauté the garlic for 1 minute. Add the spinach and tomatoes, and sauté until spinach starts to wilt. Turn off heat. Add penne and the rest of ingredients. Toss and serve.

Makes 6 servings.

Per serving: 370 calories, 13 g protein, 56 g carbohydrates, 12 g fat (3.5 g saturated), 550 mg sodium, 9 g fiber

IT TAKES STEW, BABY
(Number of Powerfoods: 5)

2 CUPS ROUGHLY TORN BABY SPINACH
½ CUP DICED RED PEPPER
1 CLOVE GARLIC, CRUSHED
1 TEASPOON OLIVE OIL
1 CAN (10.5 OUNCES) CANNELLINI BEANS, DRAINED AND RINSED
1 CUP CUBED PRECOOKED CHICKEN
½ CUP FAT-FREE REDUCED-SODIUM CHICKEN BROTH
SALT AND PEPPER

In a nonstick skillet over medium-low heat, sauté the spinach, peppers, and garlic in oil for 2 minutes, turning often. Add the beans and chicken. Sauté 1 minute more. Add the broth. Simmer for 10 minutes. Add salt and pepper.

Makes 2 servings.

Per serving: 311 calories, 27 g protein, 43 g carbohydrates, 4 g fat (0.5 g saturated), 420.5 mg sodium, 11 g fiber

MARIA'S PORTOBELLOS

2 TABLESPOONS EXTRA-VIRGIN OLIVE OIL
2 TABLESPOONS BALSAMIC VINEGAR
1 CLOVE GARLIC, MINCED
1 POUND LARGE PORTOBELLO MUSHROOMS
SALT AND PEPPER TO TASTE

Mix the oil, vinegar, and garlic in a large bowl. Add the mushrooms, letting stand for 30 minutes. Remove from the marinade and grill until golden brown. Add salt and pepper.

Makes 6 servings.

Per serving: 70 calories, 2 g protein, 5 g carbohydrates, 5 g fat (0.5 g saturated), 200 mg sodium, 1 g fiber

ABS DIET HALL OF FAME "I KNOW IT WAS YOU, ALFREDO"
(Number of Powerfoods: 6)

4 OUNCES WHOLE WHEAT SPAGHETTI
1 TEASPOON EXTRA-VIRGIN OLIVE OIL
1 CLOVE GARLIC, MINCED
¼ CUP PART-SKIM RICOTTA CHEESE
½ CUP 1 PERCENT MILK
1 CUP DRAINED CANNED SALMON
SALT AND PEPPER
2 TABLESPOONS SHREDDED PART-SKIM MOZZARELLA CHEESE

1. Cook the spaghetti according to the package directions. Drain and return to the pot.

2. Heat the oil and garlic in a large skillet over medium-low heat for 1 minute. Add the ricotta and milk and stir to combine. Add the salmon and simmer for 5 minutes. Thin with additional milk if needed. Pour over the spaghetti and season with salt and pepper. Sprinkle with the cheese.

Makes 2 servings.

Per serving: 311 calories, 27 g protein, 20 g carbohydrates, 14 g fat (6 g saturated), 543 mg sodium, 3 g fiber

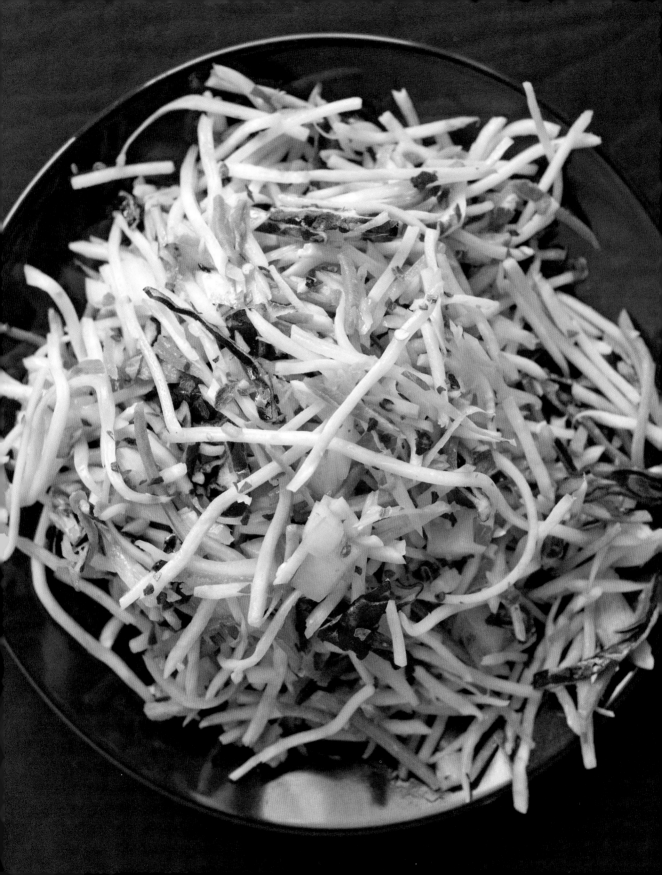

ASIAN SLAW
(Number of Powerfoods: 2)

2 CUPS PACKAGED BROCCOLI SLAW
   OR REGULAR SLAW

⅓ CUP DICED ONION

½ CUP SHREDDED CARROT

1 TABLESPOON CHOPPED CILANTRO

2 TABLESPOONS CHOPPED ALMONDS

2 TEASPOONS TOASTED SESAME OIL

1½ TABLESPOONS RICE VINEGAR

¼ TEASPOON RED-PEPPER FLAKES

Mix the slaw, onion, carrot, cilantro, and almonds in a large bowl. Mix the oil, vinegar, and pepper flakes in a small bowl. Pour over the vegetables and toss to coat.

Makes 2 servings.

Per serving: 146 calories, 6 g protein, 15 g carbohydrates, 8 g fat (1 g saturated), 48 mg sodium, 3 g fiber

BLUEBERRY-MANGO MAHI MAHI
Serve with roasted red potatoes and steamed broccoli.
(Number of Powerfoods: 3)

⅓ CUP BLUEBERRIES

⅓ CUP DICED MANGO

2 TABLESPOONS MINCED RED ONION

1 TABLESPOON MINCED CILANTRO

1 TABLESPOON LIME JUICE

½ TEASPOON MINCED JALAPEÑO PEPPER

2 TEASPOONS SUGAR

SALT AND PEPPER

1 TEASPOON EXTRA-VIRGIN OLIVE OIL

4 MAHI MAHI, RED SNAPPER, SEA BASS, OR HALIBUT FILLETS (4 OUNCES EACH)

1. Mix the blueberries, mango, onion, cilantro, lime juice, jalapeño, sugar, and ¼ teaspoon salt in a bowl. Don't worry about crushing the blueberries; you *want* to release the juice. Set aside.

2. Heat the oil in a grill pan or skillet over medium-high heat. Season the fish with salt and pepper and place, skin side down, in the pan. Cook for 4 to 5 minutes, until the skin is lightly charred and crispy. Turn and sear for another 2 to 3 minutes or until cooked through. Avoid overcooking; the fish should flake easily with a gentle touch of a fork.

3. Top each piece of fish with the blueberry mixture.

Makes 4 servings.

Per serving: 160 calories, 27 g protein, 7 g carbohydrates, 2 g fat (0 g saturated), 280 mg sodium, 1 g fiber

FOOD FACT

People who eat fish at least once a week can reduce their risk of macular degeneration—the leading cause of adult blindness—by 50 percent. The key, researchers say, may be in the omega-3 fatty acids, which may reduce inflammation in the retina.

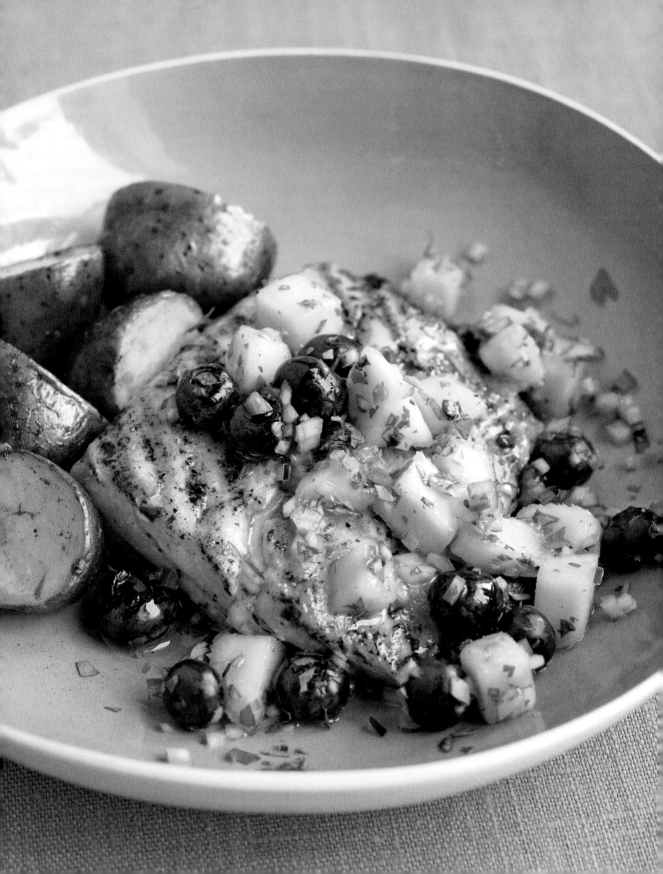

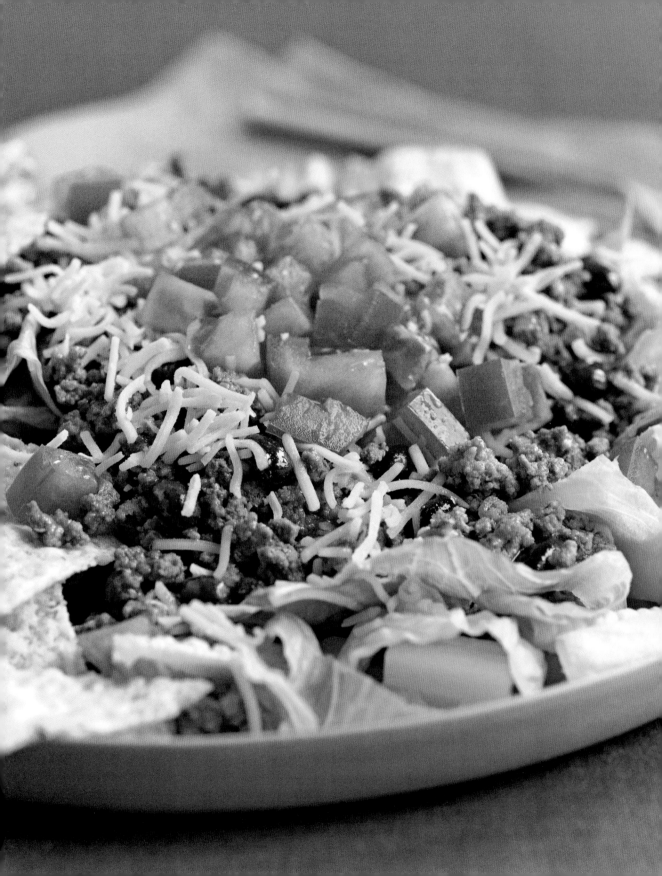

A THINNER MEXICAN DINNER
(Number of Powerfoods: 5)

FOR THE MEAT:

¾ POUND LEAN GROUND BEEF
   (90 PERCENT LEAN OR HIGHER)

2 CLOVES GARLIC, MINCED

1 CAN (15.5 OUNCES) BLACK BEANS,
   RINSED AND DRAINED

1 TABLESPOON CHILI POWDER

¼ TEASPOON CAYENNE

⅓ CUP WATER

FOR THE DRESSING:

4 MEDIUM TOMATOES, DICED

2 TABLESPOONS EXTRA-VIRGIN OLIVE OIL

2 TABLESPOONS LIME JUICE

½ TEASPOON SALT

¼ TEASPOON BLACK PEPPER

FOR THE SALAD:

2 ROMAINE LETTUCE HEARTS, CHOPPED

½ CUP SHREDDED REDUCED-FAT
   CHEDDAR CHEESE

2 OUNCES BAKED CORN TORTILLA CHIPS
   (ABOUT 32 CHIPS)

1. Heat a large skillet over medium-high heat. Add the beef and cook, breaking up the pieces with a wooden spoon, until no longer pink. Add the garlic and beans and cook for 2 minutes more. Add the chili powder, cayenne, and water and stir until well-combined and some, but not all, of the liquid has been absorbed. Remove from the heat and allow the mixture to cool slightly.

2. Mix the dressing ingredients in a bowl.

3. Divide the lettuce among dinner plates, top with the beef mixture, and sprinkle with the cheese. Spoon the dressing over each salad and crush tortilla chips on top.

Makes 4 servings.

Per serving: 440 calories, 32 g protein, 43 g carbohydrates, 19 g fat (6 g saturated), 870 mg sodium, 11 g fiber

STRIPED BASS AL FORNO
This is equally good with bluefish, mackerel, snapper, or mahi mahi.
(Number of Powerfoods: 3)

- 4 STRIPED BASS FILLETS
  SALT AND PEPPER
- 1 TABLESPOON LEMON JUICE
- 2 TABLESPOONS EXTRA-VIRGIN OLIVE OIL
- 1 TABLESPOON UNSALTED BUTTER (OPTIONAL)
- 6 PLUM TOMATOES, CHOPPED
- 1 CLOVE GARLIC, MINCED
- 16 BLACK OLIVES, PITTED AND SLICED
- 2 CUPS WHOLE GRAIN BREAD CRUMBS
  CHOPPED PARSLEY
- 16 OUNCES WHOLE WHEAT LINGUINE, COOKED

1. Place the fillets on a plate and let stand at room temperature for 20 minutes. Sprinkle lightly with salt and 1 teaspoon lemon juice. Preheat the oven to 375°F.

2. Heat 1 tablespoon oil in a small skillet over medium heat. Add the butter (if using), tomatoes, and garlic. Cook, stirring, for 2 minutes. Remove from the heat and add 2 teaspoons lemon juice and olives; season with salt and pepper.

3. Coat a large baking dish with cooking spray. Place the fillets in the dish in a single layer. Mix the bread crumbs and 1 tablespoon oil and spread on the fillets. Spoon on the tomato mixture.

4. Bake for 18 to 25 minutes or until the fish flakes easily. Sprinkle with the parsley. Serve with linguine. (If there's not enough sauce left for the pasta, repeat step 2 with new ingredients.)

Makes 6 to 8 servings, depending on the size of the fillets.

Per serving: 440 calories, 28 g protein, 62 g carbohydrates, 10 g fat (1.5 g saturated), 380 mg sodium, 9 g fiber

How to Mince an Onion

1. Cut off the ends (figure a). That will make it easy to remove the skin. **2.** Cut the onion in half and lay both halves flat side down on a cutting board so they won't roll. Hold a half firmly and make 3 or 4 horizontal cuts (figure b). **3.** Then make 5 or 6 vertical cuts. **4.** Turn the onion to make dicing cuts that are perpendicular to those you just made. With the tip of your blade planted on the board, rock the knife up and down, working it slowly across the surface of the onion (figure c).

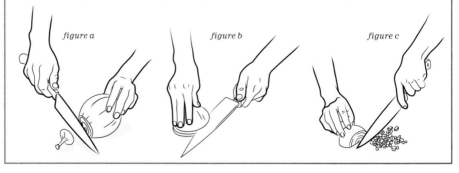

figure a   *figure b*   *figure c*

ABS DIET HALL OF FAME
THE PESTO RÉSISTANCE
(Number of Powerfoods: 5)

- 4 OUNCES WHOLE WHEAT SPAGHETTI
- 1 TABLESPOON EXTRA-VIRGIN OLIVE OIL
- ½ CUP CHOPPED WALNUTS
- 1 CLOVE GARLIC, CRUSHED
- 2 CUPS TORN BABY SPINACH LEAVES
- 1 TEASPOON DRIED BASIL
  SALT AND PEPPER
- 2 TABLESPOONS SHREDDED PART-SKIM
  MOZZARELLA CHEESE

1. Cook the spaghetti according to the package directions. Drain.

2. Heat the oil in a large nonstick skillet over medium-low heat. Add the walnuts and cook for 3 to 4 minutes, stirring frequently. Add the garlic, spinach, and basil. Cook for 3 to 5 minutes, stirring frequently. Season with salt and pepper. Add the pasta and toss to coat; sprinkle with the cheese.

Makes 2 servings.

Per serving: 335 calories, 9 g protein, 17 g carbohydrates, 28 g fat (4 g saturated), 160 mg sodium, 5 g fiber

CHILI MAC, WITH JACK
(Number of Powerfoods: 4)

- 1 POUND GROUND TURKEY
- ½ TEASPOON GARLIC POWDER
- 1 CAN (15 OUNCES) PINTO BEANS,
  RINSED AND DRAINED
- 2 CANS (14 OUNCES) DICED TOMATOES
  WITH CHILES
- 1 CUP WHOLE WHEAT ELBOW MACARONI
- 1 TABLESPOON TACO SEASONING
- ½ CUP SHREDDED REDUCED-FAT
  CHEDDAR CHEESE
- ½ CUP SHREDDED MONTEREY
  JACK CHEESE

1. Cook the turkey and garlic powder in a large skillet over medium heat, breaking up the turkey with a wooden spoon so it cooks evenly. When the turkey is no longer pink, add the beans, tomatoes with juice, macaroni, and taco seasoning. Bring to a boil.

2. Reduce the heat to low, cover and simmer for 25 minutes, stirring occasionally. During the last minute of cooking, sprinkle on the cheeses and mix so they melt into the dish.

Makes 4 servings.

Per serving: 430 calories, 35 g protein, 40 g carbohydrates, 16 g fat (6 g saturated), 1,830 mg sodium, 9 g fiber

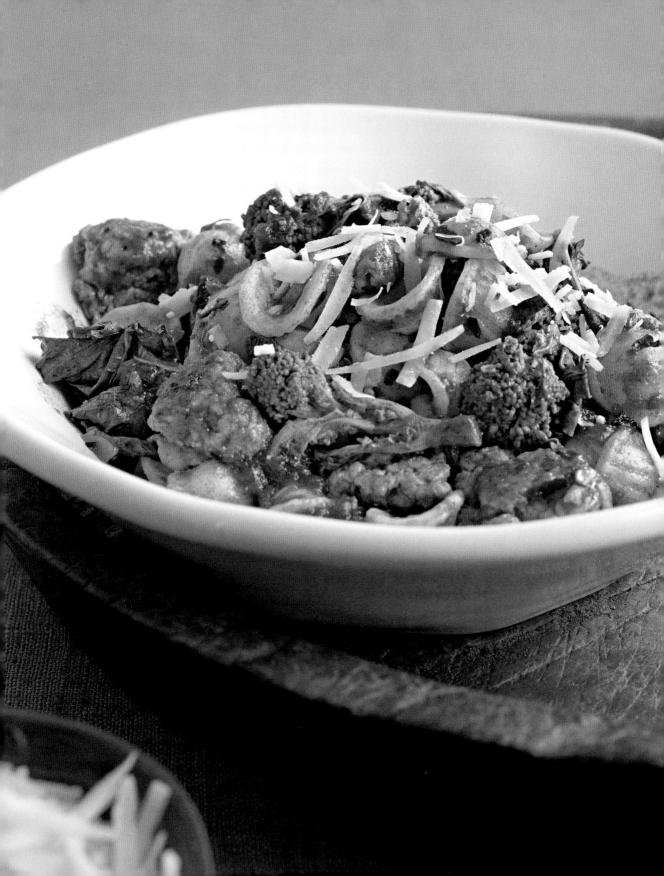

THE ITALIAN RABE
(Number of Powerfoods: 4)

1 BUNCH BROCCOLI RABE,
  TOUGH ENDS TRIMMED

12 OUNCES ORECCHIETTE PASTA

2 TABLESPOONS EXTRA-VIRGIN OLIVE OIL

1 LARGE ONION, CHOPPED

3 CLOVES GARLIC, MINCED

½ POUND HOT ITALIAN
  TURKEY SAUSAGE LINKS

2 CUPS MARINARA SAUCE

½ TEASPOON RED-PEPPER FLAKES

¼ CUP GRATED ROMANO CHEESE

¼ CUP GRATED PARMESAN CHEESE

1. Cut the broccoli rabe into 2-inch pieces. Cook the orecchiette according to the package directions; add the broccoli rabe during the last 3 minutes of cooking. Drain.

2. Heat the oil in a large skillet over medium heat. Toss in the onion and garlic and cook, stirring frequently, for 3 minutes or until translucent.

3. Remove the casing from the sausage. Add the meat to the skillet and break up the chunks with a wooden spoon. Cook for 3 minutes until nicely browned.

4. Add the pasta and broccoli rabe to the skillet and toss to combine. Stir in the marinara sauce and pepper flakes and cook until heated through. Sprinkle with the cheeses.

Makes 6 servings.

Per serving: 400 calories, 18 g protein, 52 g carbohydrates, 14 g fat (2.5 g saturated), 720 mg sodium, 4 g fiber

PROTEIN POWER BAKED ZITI

This recipe turns a carb bomb into a muscle-building feast that keeps blood sugar balanced.
(Number of Powerfoods: 3)

½ POUND WHOLE WHEAT ZITI

½ POUND BONELESS, SKINLESS CHICKEN BREASTS

1 LARGE ONION, CHOPPED

¼ CUP SUN-DRIED TOMATOES, CHOPPED

2 CLOVES GARLIC, MINCED

2 TABLESPOONS BALSAMIC VINEGAR

1 CAN (28 OUNCES) TOMATOES IN A THICK PUREE

2 TEASPOONS ITALIAN SEASONING

1 CUP SHREDDED REDUCED-FAT MOZZARELLA CHEESE

1. Coat a 2½-quart baking dish with cooking spray. Preheat the oven to 350°F.

2. Cook the ziti according to the package directions. Place in a large bowl.

3. Heat a skillet coated with cooking spray over medium heat. Add the chicken, and cook for 5 minutes or until browned on all sides. Place the cooked chicken in a bowl.

4. Spray the skillet again and cook the onion and sun-dried tomatoes for 5 minutes until soft. During the last minute, add in the garlic. Add the vinegar and cook for 3 minutes, stirring to loosen any bits that may be sticking to the pan. Stir in the canned tomatoes (including puree), Italian seasoning, and chicken. Simmer for 15 minutes. Add to the bowl with the ziti and toss.

5. Place half of the ziti mixture in the baking dish and top with ½ cup cheese. Add the remaining ziti, top with the remaining cheese, and bake for 25 minutes.

Makes 4 servings.

Per serving: 370 calories, 30 g protein, 52 g carbohydrates, 6 g fat (3 g saturated), 541 mg sodium, 7 g fiber

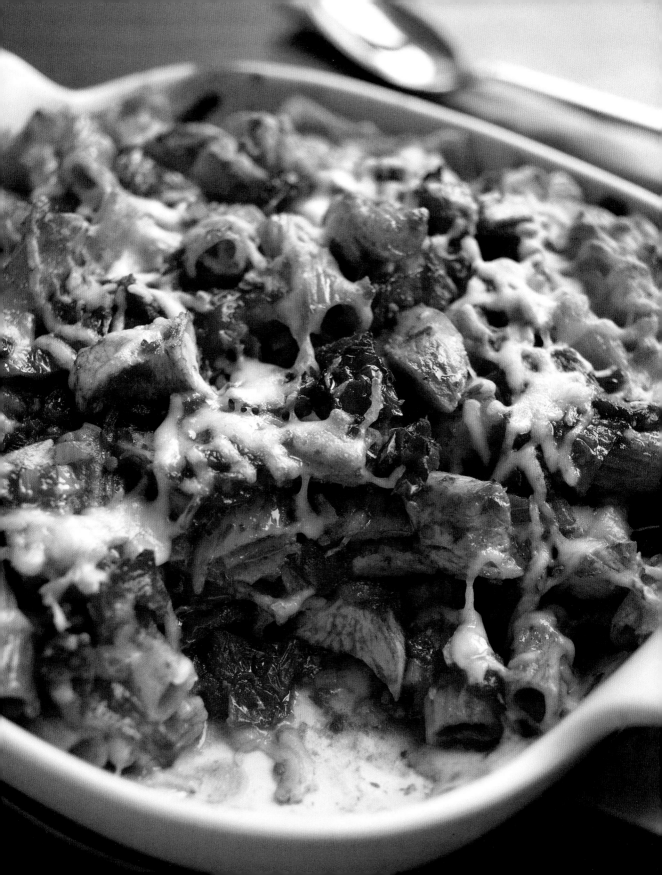

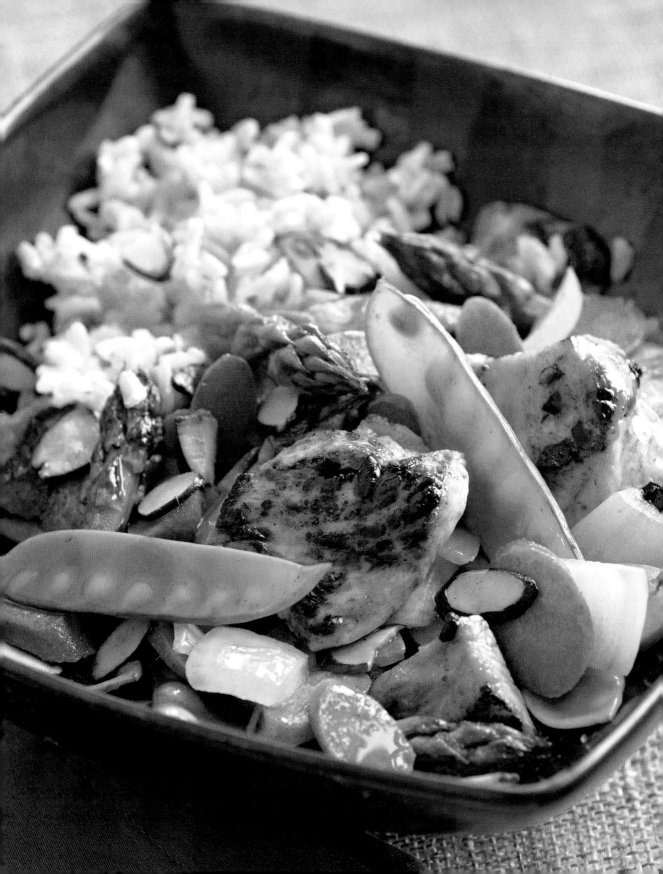

STIR-IT-UP CHICKEN AND SNOW PEAS
(Number of Powerfoods: 5)

2 TEASPOONS PEANUT OIL

¼ TEASPOON RED-PEPPER FLAKES

3 THIN-CUT BONELESS,
  SKINLESS CHICKEN BREASTS,
  CUT INTO BITE-SIZE PIECES
  OR STRIPS

⅓ CUP FROZEN SNOW PEAS

⅓ CUP ASPARAGUS TIPS

⅓ CUP THINLY SLICED CARROT

¼ MEDIUM ONION, CUT INTO
  BITE-SIZE PIECES OR STRIPS

2 TABLESPOONS SLICED ALMONDS

2 TEASPOONS REDUCED-SODIUM
  SOY SAUCE

COOKED BROWN RICE

Heat the oil and pepper flakes in
a large skillet over medium-high heat.
Add the chicken and cook for 2 to
3 minutes, stirring frequently. Add the
remaining ingredients, except rice,
and cook for another 2 to 3 minutes,
stirring often. Serve over the rice.

Makes 2 servings.

Per serving: 428 calories, 48 g protein,
20 g carbohydrates, 18 g fat
(3 g saturated), 505 mg sodium, 7 g fiber

PHILLING CHEESESTEAK TAKE 1

A healthier version of a Philadelphia institution; you won't miss the Cheez Whiz.
(Number of Powerfoods: 3)

1 CAN (8 OUNCES) TOMATO SAUCE
½ CUP LOW-SODIUM BEEF BROTH
2 TABLESPOONS WORCESTERSHIRE SAUCE
2 DASHES HOT SAUCE
3 TABLESPOONS MESQUITE SEASONING
4 THINLY SLICED TOP ROUND STEAKS (12 OUNCES)
1 GREEN BELL PEPPER, SLICED INTO STRIPS
1 ONION, SLICED
4 WHOLE GRAIN HOAGIE ROLLS
4 SLICES REDUCED-FAT PROVOLONE CHEESE
HOT BANANA PEPPER RINGS

1. Mix the tomato sauce, broth, Worcestershire, hot sauce, and 1 tablespoon of the mesquite seasoning in a bowl. Pour into a large resealable bag and add the steaks. Marinate in the refrigerator for 30 to 60 minutes.

2. Remove the steaks from the bag and shake the rest of the mesquite seasoning onto both sides of each. Reserve the marinade.

3. Coat a skillet with cooking spray and place over medium heat. Add the peppers and onions and cook, basting with a bit of the marinade, for about 5 minutes until a bit softened but not mushy.

4. Grill the steaks over medium-high heat for 3 minutes per side, basting with the marinade, until cooked to your liking. Using tongs, move the steaks to a cutting board and slice diagonally into strips. Boil the remaining marinade in a saucepan for 5 minutes.

5. Divide the meat, peppers, and onions among the rolls. Top with the cheese, a few spoonfuls of the marinade, and pepper rings.

Makes 4 servings.

Per serving: 480 calories, 41 g protein, 45 g carbohydrates, 16 g fat (7 g saturated), 1,710 mg sodium, 8 g fiber

PHILLING CHEESESTEAK TAKE 2

This one's quicker; still minus the Cheez Whiz.
(Number of Powerfoods: 3)

1 ONION, SLICED
1 RED BELL PEPPER, SLICED
1 GREEN BELL PEPPER, SLICED
⅔ CUP HOT SALSA
4 WHOLE GRAIN HOAGIE ROLLS
¾ POUND THINLY SLICED ROAST BEEF
½ CUP SHREDDED REDUCED-FAT CHEDDAR CHEESE

1. Cook the onion and bell peppers in a nonstick skillet until tender. Add the salsa and heat until warm.

2. Construct sandwiches with the rolls, roast beef, vegetables, and cheese. Warm in the microwave for 1 to 2 minutes or until the cheese starts to melt.

Makes 4 servings.

Per serving: 330 calories, 28 g protein, 41 g carbohydrates, 7 g fat (2 g saturated), 1,050 mg sodium, 7 g fiber

WHAT'S YOUR BEEF WITH BROCCOLINI?
(Number of Powerfoods: 3)

 2 TABLESPOONS OYSTER SAUCE
 2 TABLESPOONS CHOPPED FRESH GINGER
 1 TABLESPOON REDUCED-SODIUM
   SOY SAUCE
 1 TEASPOON CHILI PASTE
 1 SMALL CLOVE GARLIC, MINCED
 6 TABLESPOONS WATER
 1½ POUNDS BROCCOLINI,
   TOUGH ENDS TRIMMED
 ¾ POUND SKIRT STEAK
 2 TEASPOONS TOASTED SESAME OIL
 6 SCALLIONS, CUT INTO 1-INCH PIECES
 ⅓ CUP WALNUTS, TOASTED AND CHOPPED

1. Mix the oyster sauce, ginger, soy sauce, chili paste, garlic, and 3 tablespoons water in a small bowl.

2. Cut the broccolini into bite-size pieces. Cut the steak across the grain into thin slices.

3. Heat the oil in a large nonstick skillet over high heat. Add the broccolini and stir-fry for 3 minutes. Add 3 tablespoons water and stir-fry for 2 minutes.

4. Add the steak, scallions, and oyster sauce mixture; stir-fry until the beef is cooked through, about 2 minutes. Stir in the walnuts just before serving.

Makes 4 servings.

Per serving: 298 calories, 27 g protein, 16 g carbohydrates, 14.5 g fat (3 g saturated), 300 mg sodium, 3 g fiber

BAKED PISTACHIO CHICKEN
Serve with sautéed Swiss chard and cooked brown rice.
(Number of Powerfoods: 4; with rice and greens: 6)

 1 TABLESPOON DIJON MUSTARD
 2 TABLESPOONS EXTRA-VIRGIN
   OLIVE OIL
 2 TABLESPOONS HONEY
   SALT AND PEPPER
 1 CUP CHOPPED PISTACHIOS
 ½ CUP WHOLE GRAIN BREAD CRUMBS
 2 BONELESS, SKINLESS
   CHICKEN BREAST HALVES

1. Preheat the oven to 500°F. Coat a baking sheet with cooking spray.

2. Mix the mustard, oil, and honey in a shallow bowl; season with salt and pepper. Mix the pistachios and bread crumbs on a plate.

3. Place the chicken breasts between 2 sheets of wax paper and pound with a meat mallet to ½-inch thick. Dip the chicken in the mustard mixture to coat and then in the crumbs. Place the chicken on the baking sheet.

4. Put the baking sheet in the preheated oven. Turn the heat down to 375°F. Bake for about 20 minutes, until the chicken is no longer pink when tested with a knife.

Makes 4 servings.

Per serving (for chicken): 380 calories, 22 g protein, 25 g carbohydrates, 23 g fat (3 g saturated), 135 mg sodium, 4 g fiber

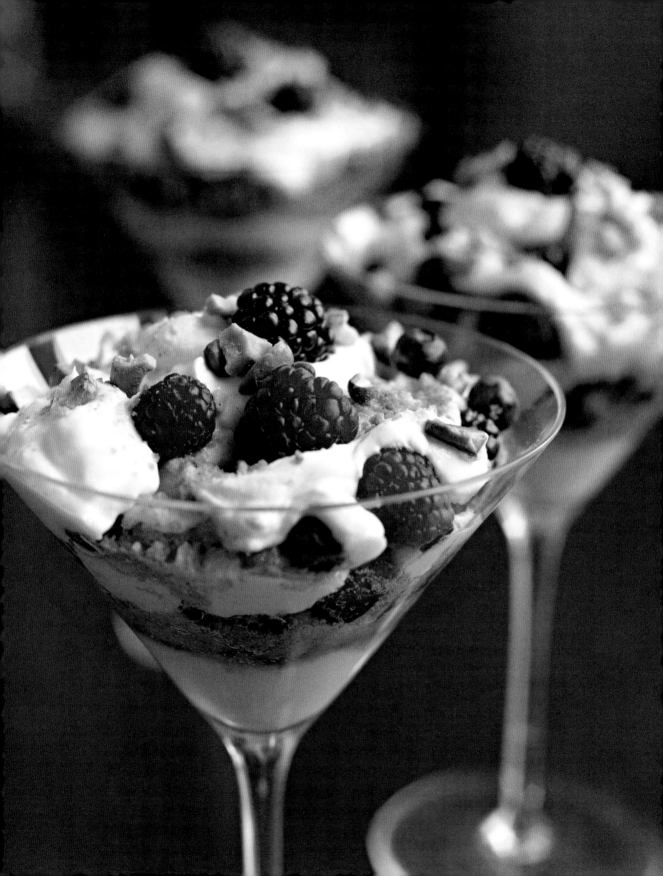

BLACKBERRY PARFAIT MARTINIS
(Number of Powerfoods: 3)

¼ CUP CRUSHED CASHEWS

2 CUPS LOW-FAT VANILLA YOGURT

1 CUP CRUSHED GRAHAM CRACKERS

½ CUP DICED STRAWBERRIES OR
TROPICAL FRUIT

2 CUPS BLACKBERRIES, RASPBERRIES,
OR BLUEBERRIES

Coat a skillet with cooking spray, add the cashews, and stir over medium heat for 2 minutes. Making thin layers, divide the yogurt, graham crackers, strawberries, and blackberries among 4 martini glasses, ending with yogurt. Top with large blackberries and the warm cashews.

Makes 4 servings.

Per serving: 210 calories, 7 g protein, 35 g carbohydrates, 6 g fat (1.5 g saturated), 90 mg sodium, 3 g fiber

WHIP-IT-GOOD BANANA SPLIT
(Number of Powerfoods: 3)

2 CUPS FAT-FREE MILK

1 PACKAGE (4 SERVINGS) JELL-O INSTANT SUGAR-FREE CHOCOLATE PUDDING MIX

2 RIPE BANANAS, SLICED

½ CUP FAT-FREE WHIPPED TOPPING

1 TABLESPOON CHOPPED PEANUTS

4 BING CHERRIES, STEM ON (OPTIONAL)

Whisk together the milk and pudding mix for about 2 minutes. Spoon half into dessert dishes. Top with bananas and then the remaining pudding. Divide the whipped topping, peanuts, and cherries (if using) among the dishes. Let stand until set, about 5 minutes.

Makes 4 servings.

Per serving: 130 calories, 5 g protein, 24 g carbohydrates, 1.5 g fat (0 g saturated), 75 mg sodium, 2 g fiber

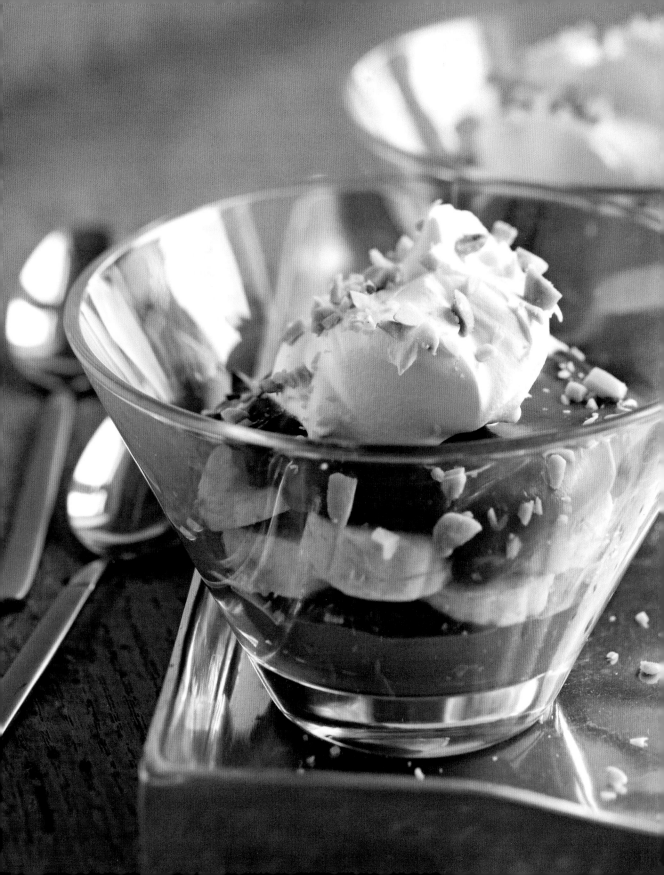

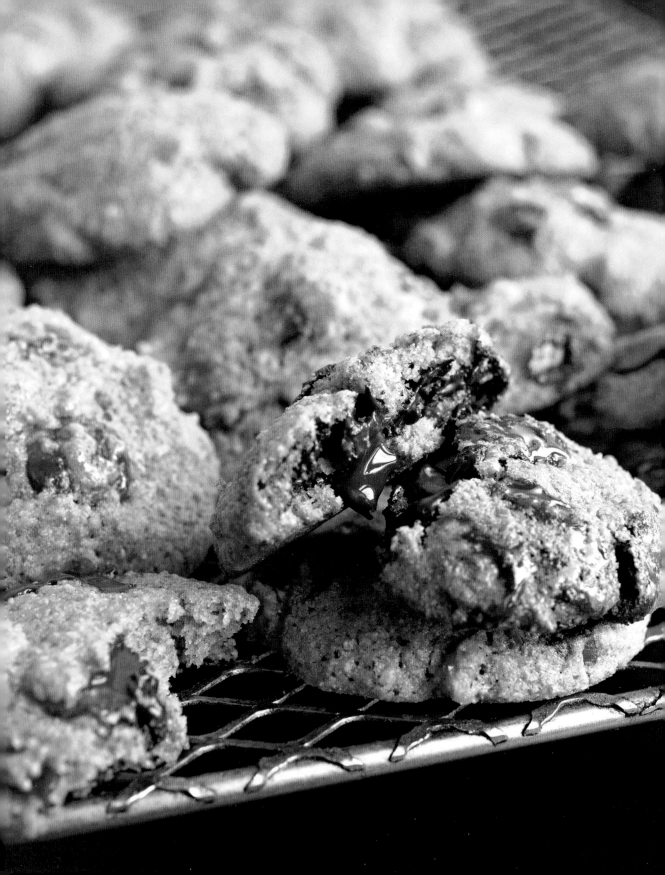

CHIPS OH BOY! COOKIES
(Number of Powerfoods: 3)

1¼ CUPS WHOLE WHEAT FLOUR
1¼ CUPS UNBLEACHED FLOUR
¾ TEASPOON BAKING SODA
½ TEASPOON SALT
½ CUP BUTTER, SOFTENED
¾ CUP GRANULATED SUGAR
¾ CUP PACKED BROWN SUGAR
2 EGGS
½ CUP UNSWEETENED APPLESAUCE
1 TEASPOON VANILLA EXTRACT
12 OUNCES DARK CHOCOLATE CHIPS
¾ CUP CHOPPED WALNUTS

1. Preheat the oven to 350°F. Coat baking sheets with cooking spray.

2. Mix the flours, baking soda, and salt in a medium bowl.

3. Beat the butter and sugars with a mixer on medium speed for about 2 minutes. Beat in the eggs, 1 at a time. Beat in the applesauce and vanilla. Add the flour mixture and mix until blended. Stir in the chocolate chips and walnuts.

4. Drop rounded tablespoons of the dough onto the baking sheets, leaving about 2 inches between cookies. Bake for 10 to 12 minutes or until golden brown. Cool on a wire rack.

Makes 36 cookies.

Per cookie: 150 calories, 2 g protein, 22 carbohydrates, 7 g fat (3.5 g saturated), 85 mg sodium, 1 g fiber

CHOCOLATE MOUSSE
(Number of Powerfoods: 1)

12 OUNCES SOFT SILKEN TOFU, DRAINED

2 TEASPOONS VANILLA EXTRACT

1 TEASPOON ALMOND EXTRACT

1 CUP SEMISWEET CHOCOLATE CHIPS, MELTED

3½ OUNCES 2 PERCENT GREEK YOGURT

Place the tofu, vanilla, and almond extract in a blender and blend until smooth. Add the chocolate and blend until smooth, scraping the sides of the container as needed. Pour into a large bowl. Fold in the yogurt until blended. Refrigerate until ready to serve.

Makes 4 servings.

Per serving: 290 calories, 10 g protein, 29 g carbohydrates, 16 g fat (8 g saturated), 15 mg sodium, 3 g fiber

CARAMEL APPLE IN A CUP
(Number of Powerfoods: 1)

1 APPLE OR ASIAN PEAR, CUBED

1 TABLESPOON SUGAR-FREE CARAMEL TOPPING

1 CONTAINER YOPLAIT LIGHT APPLE TURNOVER YOGURT

FAT-FREE WHIPPED TOPPING

Place the fruit in a fancy dessert dish. Spoon the caramel topping over it. Add the yogurt, covering all. Refrigerate for an hour, then add a spoonful of whipped topping.

Makes 1 serving.

Per serving: 300 calories, 7 g protein, 58 g carbohydrates, 6 g fat (3 g saturated), 120 mg sodium, 12 g fiber

THIS PIE'S BEEN BERRY, BERRY GOOD TO ME
(Number of Powerfoods: 1)

1 BOX (4 SERVINGS) JELL-O SUGAR-FREE STRAWBERRY GELATIN

2 TABLESPOONS CORNSTARCH

2 CUPS WATER

1 QUART STRAWBERRIES, SLICED

1 REDUCED-FAT GRAHAM CRACKER PIE CRUST (9-INCH DIAMETER)

1 CUP FAT-FREE WHIPPED TOPPING

1. Mix the gelatin and cornstarch in a medium saucepan, then stir in the water. Bring to a boil over medium heat and cook, stirring frequently, for 5 minutes, until thickened. Pour into a large heatproof bowl and allow to cool at room temperature.

2. Fold the strawberries into the gelatin. Pour into the crust. Refrigerate for at least 2 hours. Garnish with the whipped topping.

Makes 8 servings.

Per serving: 150 calories, 3 g protein, 25 g carbohydrates, 4 g fat (1 g saturated), 160 mg sodium, 1 g fiber

FIT FACT

Researchers in the UK studying cravings found that taking a 15-minute walk weakened chocolate cravings by 12 percent while staying idle intensified the desire for sweets.

ABS DIET HALL OF FAME
BANANACICLES
(Number of Powerfoods: 1)

- **4 POPSICLE STICKS**
- **2 BANANAS, PEELED AND CUT IN HALF CROSSWISE**
- **½ CUP CHOCOLATE SAUCE (THE KIND THAT FORMS A SHELL)**
- **4 TABLESPOONS UNSALTED PEANUTS, DICED**

Put a Popsicle stick into the cut end of each banana piece. Pour the chocolate sauce over the bananas until they're completely coated. Roll the chocolate-coated bananas in crushed peanuts. Freeze.

Makes 4 servings.

Per serving: 318 calories, 4 g protein, 32 g carbohydrates, 22 g fat (9 g saturated), 21 mg sodium, 4 g fiber

SOPHISTICATED S'MORES
(Number of Powerfoods: 1)

- **16 MARSHMALLOWS**
- **8 GRAHAM CRACKERS**
- **2 DARK CHOCOLATE BARS (1.5 OUNCES EACH)**
- **1 CUP BLACKBERRIES OR RASPBERRIES**

1. Cut the marshmallows in half. Break each graham cracker in half to form squares. Place 2 marshmallow halves on top of each cracker square and place as many as will fit in a toaster oven. Broil until the marshmallows turn golden brown. Break the chocolate bar into pieces.

2. Arrange the chocolate and blackberries on half of the marshmallow crackers. Cover with the remaining crackers, marshmallow side down, to make sandwiches. Squeeze gently so the hot marshmallow starts to melt the chocolate.

Makes 4 servings.

Per serving: 280 calories, 3 g protein, 50 g carbohydrates, 8 g fat (4.5 g saturated), 110 mg sodium, 4 g fiber

ABS DIET POWER TIP

I don't have to tell you that portion control is critical when it comes to cookies, but I will anyway. You can easily scarf down a meal's worth of calories with a glass of milk. So don't leave them on the counter (or risk walk-by nibbling). Have one as a treat, and put the rest out of easy reach in a high cabinet.

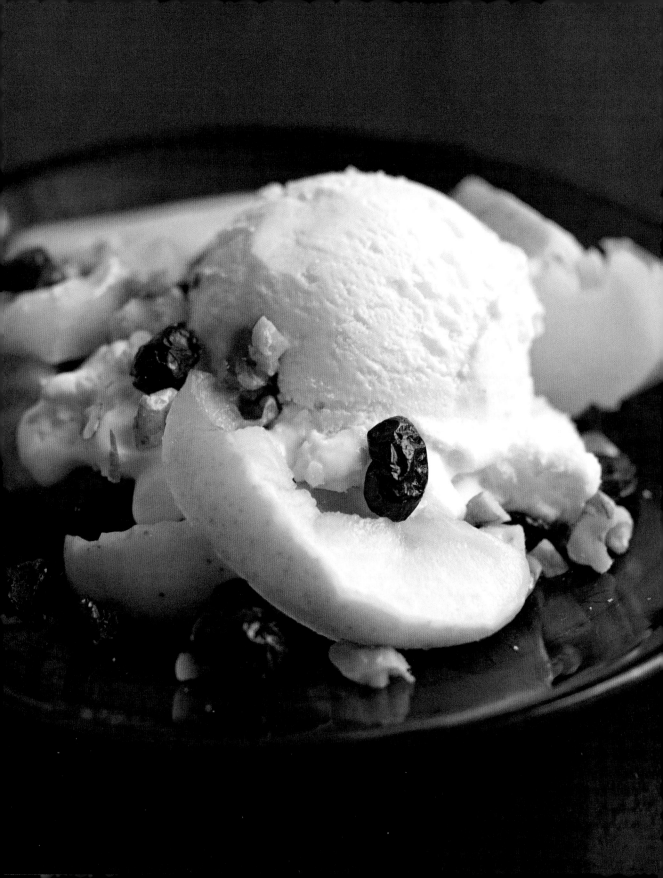

A HALF-BAKED DESSERT IDEA
(Number of Powerfoods: 3)

2 LARGE GOLDEN DELICIOUS APPLES
1 TABLESPOON LEMON JUICE
2 TABLESPOONS SUGAR
4 SCOOPS VANILLA FROZEN YOGURT
½ CUP CHOPPED WALNUTS
¼ CUP DRIED CRANBERRIES (OPTIONAL)

1. Preheat the oven to 425°F. Core the apples and cut into ½-inch slices. Place in a bowl and toss with the lemon juice. Add the sugar and toss again.

2. Dump into a baking dish. Bake for 25 minutes or until tender and golden brown. (Stir occasionally to avoid burning.)

3. Transfer to plates, top with frozen yogurt, and sprinkle with walnuts and cranberries (if using).

Makes 4 servings.

Per serving: 340 calories, 6 g protein, 51 g carbohydrates, 14 g fat (4 g saturated), 45 mg sodium, 4 g fiber

COFFEE WITH DESSERT
Make this coffee-flavored tiramisu a day ahead so it can chill properly.
(Number of Powerfoods: 2)

1½ CUPS RICOTTA CHEESE
½ CUP LIGHT CREAM CHEESE
½ CUP AND ⅓ CUP SUGAR
3 TABLESPOONS COCOA
1 EGG YOLK
1 TEASPOON VANILLA
3 EGG WHITES
¾ CUP STRONG, PREPARED COFFEE
3 TABLESPOONS
  COFFEE-FLAVORED LIQUEUR
16 LADYFINGER COOKIES

1. In a food processor, combine the ricotta cheese, cream cheese, ½ cup sugar, cocoa, egg yolk, and vanilla until smooth; transfer to a large bowl.

2. Beat the egg whites in a bowl until soft peaks form. Gradually add ⅓ cup sugar and beat until stiff peaks form. Fold the egg whites into the ricotta mixture.

3. Combine the coffee and liqueur in a small bowl.

4. Arrange half of the cookies in the bottom of a 9-inch square baking dish coated with nonstick spray. Sprinkle with half of the coffee mixture. Spread half of the ricotta mixture on top. Repeat one more layer. Cover and chill overnight.

Makes 16 servings.

Per serving: 150 calories, 6 g protein, 21 g carbohydrates, 5 g fat (2 g saturated), 102 mg sodium, 0 g fiber

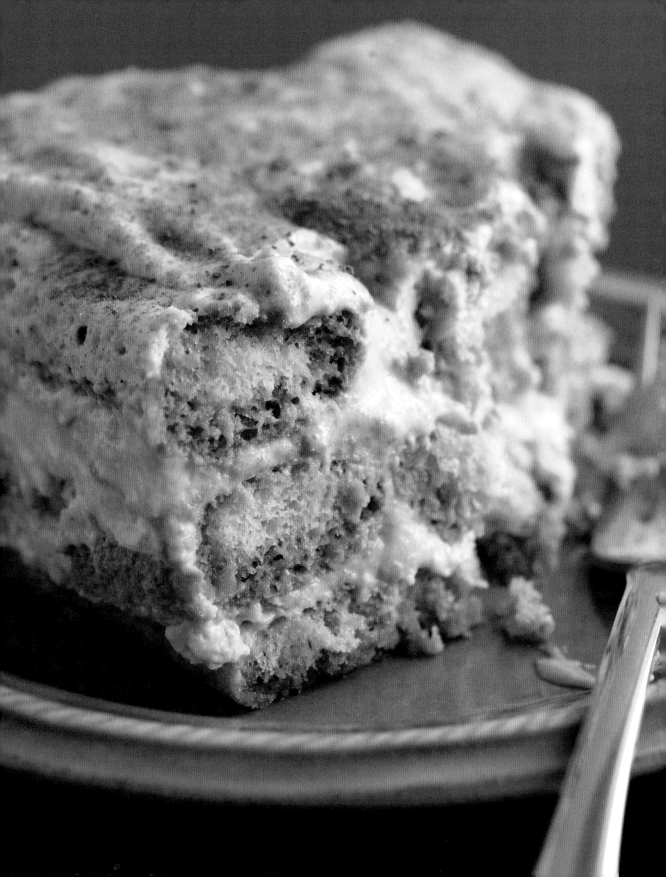

UNCLE CLEM'S COWBOY COBBLER
(Number of Powerfoods: 2)

⅓ CUP BUTTER, SOFTENED

1 CAN (29 OUNCES) UNSWEETENED PEACH SLICES, DRAINED

⅔ CUP PACKED BROWN SUGAR

½ CUP WHOLE WHEAT FLOUR

½ CUP ROLLED OATS

¾ TEASPOON GROUND CINNAMON

¾ TEASPOON GROUND NUTMEG

1. Preheat the oven to 375°F. Spread the butter in an 8-by-8-inch baking dish. Add the peaches in an even layer.

2. Mix the sugar, flour, oats, cinnamon, and nutmeg and sprinkle over the peaches.

Bake for 30 minutes, until brown.

Makes 8 servings.

Per serving: 210 calories, 2 g protein, 33 g carbohydrates, 8 g fat (5 g saturated), 10 mg sodium, 3 g fiber

JAMMED BERRY CHEESECAKE
(Number of Powerfoods: 3)

1 8-OUNCE PACKAGE FAT-FREE CREAM CHEESE

2 8-OUNCE PACKAGES REDUCED-FAT CREAM CHEESE

1 CUP SUGAR

½ CUP SPLENDA

2 TABLESPOONS ALL-PURPOSE FLOUR

1 TEASPOON VANILLA EXTRACT

2 EGGS

2 EGG WHITES

2 CUPS FRESH RASPBERRIES

1 REDUCED-FAT GRAHAM CRACKER CRUST (9-INCH DIAMETER)

1. Preheat the oven to 350°F.

2. Dump the cream cheeses, sugar, Splenda, flour, and vanilla in a large bowl. Using an electric mixer, combine the ingredients. Then add all the eggs and whip until the mixture is smooth.

3. In a medium bowl, crush the raspberries with a fork. Spoon half of the crushed berries into the cream cheese filling and mix with a spoon. Then spoon the cheesecake mixture into the pie crust. Top the mixture with the remaining crushed berries and smooth the top with a small baking spatula.

4. Place on a baking sheet and bake for 1 hour, or until a toothpick poked into the center comes out clean. Let cool out of the oven, then cover and refrigerate for 4 hours before serving.

Makes 16 servings.

Per serving: 140 calories, 7 g protein, 13 g carbohydrates, 7 g fat (4 g saturated), 216 mg sodium, 1.5 g fiber

ABS DIET POWER TIP

Drink mint tea with your dessert. It contains the powerful antioxidant hesperidin, which reduces the inflammation and oxidative stress associated with diabetes by 52 percent, according to a study at the University of Buffalo.

MUSCLE MUFFINS
(Number of Powerfoods: 3)

1 BANANA, MASHED

1 APPLE, SHREDDED

½ CUP UNSWEETENED APPLESAUCE

¼ CUP CHOPPED WALNUTS

1 SCOOP VANILLA WHEY
PROTEIN POWDER

1 CUP WHOLE GRAIN PASTRY FLOUR

3 TABLESPOONS BROWN SUGAR

2 TEASPOONS BAKING POWDER

1. Preheat the oven to 350°F.
Coat a nonstick muffin pan with
cooking spray.

2. Mix all the ingredients. Spoon into
the muffin cups. Bake for 20 minutes or
until a toothpick inserted into the
center of a muffin comes out clean.

Makes 12 muffins.

Per muffin: 90 calories, 3 g protein,
15 g carbohydrates, 2 g fat
(0 g saturated), 85 mg sodium, 2 g fiber

GRILLED DESSERT KEBOBS
(Number of Powerfoods: 2)

2 TABLESPOONS HONEY

1 TABLESPOON BROWN SUGAR

1 TEASPOON LEMON JUICE

¼ TEASPOON GROUND CINNAMON

1 TEASPOON WATER

12 STRAWBERRIES

2 RIPE NECTARINES, EACH CUT INTO
6 WEDGES

12 1-INCH-THICK BANANA SLICES

2 RIPE PLUMS, EACH CUT INTO
6 WEDGES

2 1½-INCH-THICK SLICES OF ANGEL FOOD
CAKE, EACH CUT INTO 6 CUBES

1 CUP PLAIN LOW-FAT YOGURT

1. Soak six 8-inch to 10-inch wooden
skewers in water for 30 minutes.
(Or use metal skewers.)

2. Mix the honey, brown sugar,
lemon juice, cinnamon, and water in
a small bowl.

3. Thread the fruit and cake cubes onto
the skewers in alternating fashion.
Brush the kebabs with the honey-sugar
mixture. Save any extra.

4. Spray cooking oil on a grill. Place the
kebabs on the grate over medium-hot
heat. Grill for about 5 minutes, turning
twice, until the fruit is heated and the
cake is slightly browned.

5. Combine the remaining honey
mixture with the yogurt and drizzle
over the kebabs.

Makes 6 servings.

Per serving: 142 calories, 2 g protein,
34 g carbohydrates, 1 g fat
(0 g saturated), 14 mg sodium, 2 g fiber

ABS DIET POWER TIP

You can do
without sugary
juices and sodas.
For a flavorful
and refreshing
beverage, squeeze
wedges of lemon,
lime, tangerine, or
pink grapefruit
into a pitcher of ice
water. If you plan
ahead, you can
make the ice cubes
using water with
a splash of 100
percent white
grape or apple
juice and bits of
real fruit. Stir in
some fresh mint or
grated ginger to
complete this low-
calorie, virgin
cocktail.

APPENDIX A
The New Abs Diet Cookbook Two-Week Meal Plan

WHAT'S FOR DINNER? Easy. Just follow the sample 14-day meal plan below. It's a no-bean-sprout zone, filled with some of the delicious recipes found in this book. The meals are based on the 12 Abs Diet Powerfoods—those nutritionally dense, fiber- and protein-rich staples that make losing weight delicious. Included are approximate calorie counts for those who wish to keep track. Note: Additional side dishes, snacks, and beverages will increase total calories.

SUNDAY
Day 1

Breakfast: 2 fried eggs with God-Didn't-Make-Little-Green-Apples Home Fries (page 66)

Snack 1: 1 cup low-fat yogurt

Lunch: It's a Lentil soup (page 172), hunk of crusty bread

Snack 2: Rip-Roarin' Roasted Red Pepper Sauce (page 114) with 5 homemade whole wheat pita wedges; unsweetened iced tea

Dinner: Dr. Flank 'N' Stein's Monster with sautéed spinach (page 188) and Potato Salad with Warm Bacon Dressing (page 197)

Dessert: Whip-It-Good Banana Split (page 234)

TOTAL CALORIES: 1,575

MONDAY
Day 2

Breakfast: The Ultimate Power Breakfast (page 86)

Snack 1: Mango Tango smoothie (page 103)

Lunch: The Muscle Maker salad using leftover flank steak from Sunday dinner (page 136)

Snack 2: 1 stick string mozzarella cheese, 1 medium apple

Dinner: The Pesto Résistance (page 223)

Snack 3 (optional): 2 cups popcorn sprinkled with Old Bay Seasoning and cayenne pepper

TOTAL CALORIES: 1,513

TUESDAY
Day 3

Breakfast: The Kitchen Sink breakfast smoothie (page 104)

Snack 1: 1 hard-cooked egg, 7 baby carrots

Lunch: Turkey and Swiss cheese sandwich with mustard on whole wheat pita bread, 1 pretzel rod, 1 medium pear

Snack 2: 1 ounce almonds, 1 cup 1 percent chocolate milk

Dinner: The Official Abs Diet Burger (page 195), *Men's Health* Spicy Oven Fries (page 108), and dinner salad with 1 tablespoon olive oil and vinegar dressing

Snack 3 or Dessert (optional): Your choice.

TOTAL CALORIES: 1,688

WEDNESDAY
Day 4

Breakfast: Breakfast Dogs (page 68)

Snack 1: 1 medium wedge cantaloupe; one 5.3-ounce container Greek yogurt

Lunch: Go Fig-Ure Panini (page 141)

Snack 2: 2 tablespoons Take a Quick Dip (page 117), 5 ounces broccoli florets

Dinner: Stir-It-Up Chicken and Snow Peas (page 229)

Dessert (optional): 2 Chips Oh Boy! Cookies (page 237), 8 ounces fat-free milk

TOTAL CALORIES: 1,798

THURSDAY
Day 5

Breakfast: Liquid Sandwich smoothie (page 97)

Snack 1: 1 bowl oatmeal with raisins

Lunch: Man-Can-Live-Without-Bread Chicken Salad Sandwich (page 145)

Snack 2: 1½ cups berries, ¾ cup low-fat ice cream

Dinner: Protein Power Baked Ziti (page 226), small dinner salad with Romaine lettuce and cherry tomatoes, olive oil and balsamic vinegar

Snack 3: Flower Power smoothie (page 105)

TOTAL CALORIES: 1,745

FRIDAY
Day 6

Breakfast: A Guac in the Park Breakfast Burrito (page 88)

Snack 1: 1 medium pear

Lunch: Roast Beef and Horseradish Wrap (page 133)

Snack 2: Tailgate Party Nut Mix (page 113)

Dinner: Walk-the-Plank Salmon with Grilled Pineapple and Asparagus (pages 192 and 203)

Dessert: Blackberry Parfait Martinis (page 233)

TOTAL CALORIES: 1,686

SATURDAY
Day 7

Breakfast: Flapjacks with Chocolate Chips (page 83)

Snack 1: Halle Berries Smoothie (make extra to save for an evening snack)(page 95)

Lunch: Can't Beet This Salad (page 167)

Snack 2: Guiltless Tailgate Wings (page 117)

Dinner: Cheat Meal! This is your chance to eat whatever you've been craving: beer and burgers, wine and cheese, Chinese food, whatever. You've been doing great; have a favorite to celebrate.

TOTAL CALORIES: Fuggetaboutit. Today's your cheat meal day.

SUNDAY
Day 8

Breakfast: Overtime Oats (page 69)

Snack 1: El Desayuno Wrap (page 71)

Lunch: Reuben Made Betta (page 135)

Snack 2: Hummus a Tuna (page 111)

Dinner: Chicken Soup for the Bowl (page 168)

Snack 3: A Half-Baked Dessert Idea (page 241)

TOTAL CALORIES: 1,760

MONDAY
Day 9

Breakfast: The Kitchen Sink (page 104)

Snack 1: 1 tablespoon peanut butter, raw vegetable sticks (as much as you like)

Lunch: Turkey or roast beef sandwich on whole grain bread, 1 cup 1 percent milk, 1 apple

Snack 2: 1 ounce almonds, 1½ cups berries

Dinner: Baked Pistachio Chicken (page 231)

Snack 3: Light popcorn sprinkled with Parmesan cheese

TOTAL CALORIES: 1,513

TUESDAY
Day 10

Breakfast: Eggs Beneficial Breakfast Sandwich (page 75)

Snack 1: Guac 'n' Roll (page 68)

Lunch: Popeye and Olive Oil Salad (page 128)

Snack 2: 1 cup low-fat yogurt; 1 ounce pistachios

Dinner: The Weight-Loss Burger (page 202)

Snack 3: 4 strawberries, 1 square dark chocolate

TOTAL CALORIES: 1,669

WEDNESDAY
Day 11

Breakfast: Veggie Sausage Wrap (page 68)

Snack 1: String cheese stick, 1 medium apple

Lunch: All 'Choked Up salad (page 154)

Snack 2: Chocolate Pudding Milk Shake (page 104)

Dinner: Don't Tell Mom It's Not Meat Loaf (page 140); The Monster Mash (page 165)

Dessert: Bananacicles (page 239)

TOTAL CALORIES: 1,633

THURSDAY
Day 12

Breakfast: Almond Joy smoothie (page 97)

Snack 1: 1 slice Swiss cheese rolled up with 3 slices turkey deli meat

Lunch: ½ leftover meat loaf sandwich with ketchup on whole grain bread

Snack 2: Low-fat ice cream sandwich

Dinner: Son-of-a-Gun Stew (page 212)

Dessert: Caramel Apple in a Cup (page 238)

TOTAL CALORIES: 1,693

FRIDAY
Day 13

Breakfast: Dinner-for-Breakfast Burrito (page 82)

Snack 1: ½ cup high-fiber cereal, ½ cup fat-free milk

Lunch: Eat-the-Bowl Bean Salsa (page 132)

Snack 2: Mango Tango smoothie (page 103)

Dinner: Cheat Meal! Whatever you crave. Go for it!

TOTAL CALORIES: No counting. It's your cheat meal day.

SATURDAY
Day 14

Breakfast: Grilled Banana Sandwiches (page 85)

Snack 1: The Immune Booster smoothie (page 103)

Lunch: Can't Beet This Salad (page 167)

Snack 2: 1 ounce Cheddar cheese; 5 wheat crackers

Dinner: The Italian Rabe (page 225)

Dessert: Coffee with Dessert (coffee-flavored tiramisu) (page 242)

TOTAL CALORIES: 1,604 (or about 1,800 if you go for another half serving of The Italian Rabe)

APPENDIX B

The New Abs Diet Exercise Plan

IN THE PREVIOUS Abs Diet books, I recommend that people new to the system get the food part of the program figured out before jumping into the workout. Concentrate on acclimating your body to eating the powerfoods six times a day. Take two weeks getting used to the diet, and then add the exercise program. If you've been using this cookbook for a few weeks, you're ready to turbocharge the Abs Diet with exercise.

The Abs Diet Workout is a fairly simple routine that's ideal for beginners. It's not intimidating. You don't have to belong to a gym to do it. The exercises can be done in the privacy of your own home with very little equipment. Optional, but recommended, gear includes a flat bench, one or two pairs of medium-weight dumbbells (5 to 25 pounds for someone with some experience lifting weights; lighter for beginners), running shoes, and a Swiss ball, also called a stability ball. That's it.

The Abs Diet workout focuses on three effective fat-burning components:

1. Strength training. Three times a week. You'll target the big muscle groups of the body: the legs, the back and chest, and shoulders because that's where you can build the most muscle in the least amount of time. I'm not talking about turning you into the next Hulk. Rather, I'm talking lean, strong, sexy muscle. Each pound of lean muscle on your body uses up to 50 calories a day just to maintain itself. So by adding just 3 pounds of muscle, you'll burn up to an extra 150 calories a day without lifting a finger. What's more, the workout is planned in circuit-training fashion. You'll perform different exercises one after another, with little rest. This has two big benefits: It keeps your workouts brief so you can get on with life; and by keeping your heart rate elevated with speedy moves, you'll maximize your fat burn and gain cardiovascular benefits, too.

2. Additional cardiovascular exercise. On non-strength-training days, you can swim, run, cycle, walk, or use cardio machines. I recommend one high-intensity interval-training workout one day a week. Studies show that intervals are far more effective at burning calories than long slow cardio workouts.

3. Abs exercise. Twice a week. I recommend doing them before your strength training or interval workouts. These moves help tone and strengthen the core muscles that support your spine—and that look so good at the beach when they are sculpted into six hard, little ripples over your midsection.

You'll find detailed instructions for performing all these workouts and individual moves in the books *The New Abs Diet* and *The New Abs Diet for Women*. But if you want to get started in a light strength-training program immediately, I recommend you ease into exercise with this workout three times a week: Do three sets of pushups and three sets of squats with no weights. Both exercises use your body weight as resistance and will get your body accustomed to a strength-training program. Alternate the exercises. Do 8 to 10 repetitions of pushups followed by 15 to 20 repetitions of squats. Then repeat the sequence twice more. You can rest for 30 seconds to a minute between exercises. When that workout becomes too easy, increase the repetitions of pushups and hold on to some form of weight for the squats. Light dumbbells are best, but you can also use cans of beans or jugs of water for resistance. This light workout, especially in combination with 30 minutes of brisk walking, will really fire up your fat burners. Then, when you are ready, move on to the strength, interval, and core workouts outlined in *The New Abs Diet* books and other workouts at www.menshealth.com/abs-diet-club.

Nutritional Values of Common Foods

THIS NEW TREND toward low-carb diets has a lot of us eating plenty of fat and protein. But many of us are missing out on the valuable micronutrients found in whole grains, fruits, vegetables, and other foods that are verboten on a low-carb diet.

It might seem easier to ensure your daily value of nutrients by popping a multivitamin instead of eating a balanced diet. But there are two problems with nutrition that comes in a plastic container: First, multivitamins have no fiber, so this critical nutrient is missing if all you do is pop a pill for protection. Second, foods are loaded with plenty of nutrients beyond the standard vitamins C and E—and the importance of many of these nutrients, called phytochemicals, is only now being understood. "In a balanced diet, there are thousands of antioxidants. In pill form, you're just getting a few out of the thousands," says Edgar Miller, MD, PhD, of Johns Hopkins University in Baltimore.

To see how nutritionally complete your diet is, refer to the following chart for each food's vitamin and mineral values, and tally your total intake. If you come up short of the Recommended Dietary Allowances (RDAs) for men and women, don't worry. Just eat more foods high in whatever vitamins or minerals you're lacking, and take a multivitamin/mineral supplement each day.

	VITAMIN A (MCG)	VITAMIN B1 (THIAMIN) (MG)	VITAMIN B6 (MG)	FOLATE (MCG)	VITAMIN C (MG)
RDA (men/women)	**900/700**	**1.2/1.1**	**1.3/1.3**	**400/400**	**95/75**
Almonds (1 ounce)	0	0.05	0.03	11	0
Apple (1 medium)	8	0.02	0.06	4	6
Apricot (1)	67	0.01	0.02	3	3.50
Artichoke (1 medium)	0	0.10	0.15	87	15
Asparagus (1 medium spear)	12	0.02	0.01	8	1
Avocado (1)	122	0.20	0.60	124	16
Bacon (3 slices)	0	0.08	0.07	0.40	0
Bagel (4 inches)	0	0.15	0.05	20	0
Banana (1 medium)	7	0.04	0.40	24	10
Beans, baked (1 cup)	13	0.40	0.34	61	8
Beans, black (1 cup cooked)	1	0.40	0.12	256	0
Beans, kidney (1 cup cooked)	0	0.28	0.21	230	2
Beans, lima (½ cup cooked)	32	0.12	0.16	22	9
Beans, navy (1 cup cooked)	0.36	0.40	0.30	255	1.64
Beans, pinto (1 cup cooked)	0	0.17	0.16	294	1.37
Beans, refried (1 cup)	0	0.07	0.36	28	15
Beans, white (1 cup cooked)	0	0.20	0.17	145	0
Beef, ground lean (3 ounces)	0	0.06	0.24	7	0
Beer (12 ounces)	0	0.02	0.18	21	0
Beets (½ cup)	3	0.02	0.05	74	3
Blueberries (1 pint)	17	0.11	0.15	17	28
Bran, wheat (1 cup)	0	0.14	0.35	14	0
Bread, rye (1 slice)	0.26	0.14	0.02	35	0.13
Bread, white (1 slice)	0	0.11	0.02	28	0
Bread, whole grain (1 slice)	0	0.11	0.10	30	0.08
Breakfast sandwich, fast-food (bacon, egg, and cheese)	0	0.53	0.16	73	2
Brussels sprouts (½ cup)	60	0.08	0.14	47	48

VITAMIN E (MG)	CALCIUM (MG)	MAGNESIUM (MG)	POTASSIUM (MG)	SELENIUM (MCG)	ZINC (MG)	CALORIES
15/15	**1,000/1,000**	**420/320**	**4,700/4,700**	**55/55**	**11/8**	**–**
6	71	86	180	0	1	170
0.25	8	7	148	0	0.06	80
0.30	5	3.50	90	0.03	0.07	20
0.24	56	77	474	0.26	0.60	25
0.18	4	2	32	0.37	0.10	5
3	22	78	1,204	0.80	0.84	25
0.06	2	6	107	12	0.70	110
0.04	16	26	90	28	1	247
0.12	6	32	422	1	0.20	110
1.35	127	81	752	12	4	239
0.14	46	120	610	2	1.90	240
0.05	62	74	717	2	1.80	260
0.12	27	63	485	1.70	0.70	229
0.73	127	107	670	11	1.90	255
1.61	72	70	495	19	1.70	245
0	88	83	675	3	3	240
1.74	161	113	1,004	2.30	2.50	249
0.15	7	19	265	0	4	185
0	18	21	89	2.50	0.04	153
0.03	111	16	221	0.5	0.24	29
1.65	17	17	223	0.3	0.50	165
0.54	26	220	426	28	3	120
0.11	23	13	53	10	0.36	83
0.06	38	6	25	4.30	0.20	67
0.09	24	14	53	8	0.30	65
0.60	160	24	211	36.0	2	441
0.34	28	16	247	1.17	0.26	28

	VITAMIN A (MCG)	VITAMIN B1 (THIAMIN) (MG)	VITAMIN B6 (MG)	FOLATE (MCG)	VITAMIN C (MG)
RDA (men/women)	**900/700**	**1.2/1.1**	**1.3/1.3**	**400/400**	**95/75**
Cake, coffee (1 piece)	20	0.10	0.03	27	0.11
Cake, frosted (1 piece)	10	0.01	0.02	7	0.04
Canadian bacon (2 slices)	0	0.40	0.20	2	0
Candy, nonchocolate (1 package)	0	0	0	0	0
Cantaloupe (1 medium wedge)	345	0.04	0.07	21	37
Carrot (1)	734	0.04	0.08	12	4
Cauliflower (1 cup)	2	0.06	0.22	57	46
Celery (1 cup, strips)	55	0.03	0.10	45	4
Cereal, whole grain, with raisins (½ cup)	3	0.16	0.10	22	0.55
Cheddar cheese (1 slice)	75	0.01	0.2	5	0
Chef's salad with no dressing (1½ cups)	146	0.40	0.40	101	16
Cherries, sweet, raw (1 cup)	30	0.07	0.05	5.80	10
Chicken, skinless (½ breast)	4	0.04	0.32	2	0.71
Chickpeas (1 cup cooked)	4	0.19	0.22	282	2
Chili with beans (1 cup)	87	0.12	0.30	59	4
Chips, potato, light (1 ounce)	0	0.05	0.22	8	3.40
Chocolate (1.45 ounces)	20	0.05	0.01	5	0
Cinnamon bun (1)	0	0.12	0	17	0.06
Citrus fruits and frozen concentrate juices (12 ounces)	7	0.17	0.30	31	324
Clams, fried (¾ cup)	101	0.11	0.07	41	11.25
Coffee (1 cup)	0	0	0	5	0
Collards (1 cup cooked)	0.08	0.8	0.24	177	35
Cookie, chocolate chip (1)	0.04	0.01	0.01	0.90	0
Corn (1 cup)	0.26	0.06	0.16	115	12
Cottage cheese, low-fat (1 cup)	25	0.05	0.15	27	0
Crackers (12)	0	0.17	0	0	0
Cranberry juice cocktail (1 cup)	1	0.02	0.05	0	90

VITAMIN E (MG)	CALCIUM (MG)	MAGNESIUM (MG)	POTASSIUM (MG)	SELENIUM (MCG)	ZINC (MG)	CALORIES
15/15	**1,000/1,000**	**420/320**	**4,700/4,700**	**55/55**	**11/8**	–
0.11	76	10	63	9	0.25	180
0	18	14	84	1.40	0.30	239
0.16	5	10	181	11	0.80	137
0	0	0	0	0	0	230
0.05	9	12	272	0.40	0.18	24
0.40	20	7	195	0.06	0.15	35
0.08	22	15	303	0.60	0.30	25
0.33	50	14	322	0.50	0.16	17
0.40	33	70	207	10	1	195
0.08	204	8	28	4	0.90	114
0	235	49	401	37	3	267
0.20	21	16	325	0.90	0.09	90
0.08	6.50	16	150	11	0.50	130
0.60	80	79	477	6	2.50	269
1.46	120	115	934	3	5	220
0.62	10	18	285	2	0.17	142
0.83	78	26	153	2	0.83	230
0.48	10	3.60	19	5	0.10	418
0.24	85	68	1,336	1	0.41	186
0	71	16	366	33	1.60	560
0.05	2	5	114	0	0.02	2
1.67	266	38	220	1	0.50	61
0.26	2.50	3	14	0	0.06	63
0.15	8	44	343	1.54	1.36	120
0.02	138	11	194	20	.86	180
0	28	12	48	2.40	0.20	155
0	8	5	46	0	0.18	137

	VITAMIN A (MCG)	VITAMIN B1 (THIAMIN) (MG)	VITAMIN B6 (MG)	FOLATE (MCG)	VITAMIN C (MG)
RDA (men/women)	**900/700**	**1.2/1.1**	**1.3/1.3**	**400/400**	**95/75**
Cream cheese (1 tablespoon)	53	0	0	2	0
Cucumber with peel (½ cup)	10	0.01	0.02	7	2.76
Doughnut (1)	17	0.10	0.03	24	0.09
Egg, whole (1 large)	84	0.03	0.06	22	0
Eggplant (1 cup)	4	0.08	0.09	14	1
English muffin, whole wheat (1)	0.09	0.25	0.05	36	0
Fig bar cookies (2 bars)	3	0.05	0.02	11	0.10
Fish, white (1 fillet)	60	0.26	0.50	26	0
French fries (10)	0	0.07	0.16	8	6
Fruit, dried (1 ounce)	208	0.01	0.05	1.10	1
Fruit juice, unsweetened (1 cup)	0	0.02	0.06	35	40
Garlic (1 clove)	0	0	0.04	0.09	0.90
Graham cracker (1 large rectangular piece)	0	0.03	0.01	6	0
Granola bar (1)	2	0.06	0.02	6	0.22
Grape juice (1 cup)	1	0.07	0.16	8	0.25
Ham (1 slice)	0	0.20	0.10	1	0
Hamburger, fast-food, with condiments and vegetables (1)	4	0.30	0.12	52	2
Hot dog, fast-food (1)	0	0.44	0.09	85	0.09
Ice cream (1 serving)	6	0.03	0.04	11	0.46
Jam or preserves (1 tablespoon)	0.20	0.0	0	2	2
Kale (1 cup)	955	0.07	0.11	18	33
Ketchup (1 tablespoon)	7	0	0.02	2	2
Kiwifruit (1 medium)	3	0.02	0.07	19	70
Lasagna, meat (7 ounces)	61	0.19	0.20	16	12
Lentils (1 cup cooked)	4.75	0.33	0.35	358	0.22
Lettuce, iceberg (1 cup)	8	0.02	0.03	31	2
Lettuce, romaine (½ cup)	81	0.02	0.02	38	7
Liver, beef (3 ounces)	8,042	0.16	0.86	215	1.62

VITAMIN E (MG)	CALCIUM (MG)	MAGNESIUM (MG)	POTASSIUM (MG)	SELENIUM (MCG)	ZINC (MG)	CALORIES
15/15	**1,000/1,000**	**420/320**	**4,700/4,700**	**55/55**	**11/8**	**–**
0.04	12	1	17	0.40	0.10	51
0	7	6	75	0	0.10	8
0.90	21	9	60	4	0.30	230
0.50	25	5	63	15	0.50	74
0.40	6	11	122	0.10	0.12	35
0.26	101	21	106	17	0.61	134
0.21	20	9	66	1	0.12	111
0.39	51	65	625	25	2	168
0.12	4	11	211	0.20	0.20	100
0.31	11.82	11.13	226	0	0.14	69
0.20	160	9	154	0	0.20	117
0	5	0.75	12	0.40	0	4
0	3	4	19	1	0.10	59
0.05	15	24	82	4	0.50	117
0.62	23	25	334	0.25	0.13	154
0.32	2	5	94	6	0.50	30
0	126	23	251	20	2	512
.10	108	27	190	29	2	242
0	72	19	164	1.65	0.40	133
0	4	0.80	15	.40	0	56
1	180	23	417	1.17	0.23	39
0.20	3	3	57	0.04	0	15
1	26	13	237	0.15	0.10	50
0.94	220	41	372	28	3	318
2.97	37	71	731	5.54	2.51	230
0.02	11	4	84	0.28	0.10	8
0.04	9	4	69	0.10	0.06	5
0.43	5	18	300	31	4.50	162

	VITAMIN A (MCG)	VITAMIN B1 (THIAMIN) (MG)	VITAMIN B6 (MG)	FOLATE (MCG)	VITAMIN C (MG)
RDA (men/women)	**900/700**	**1.2/1.1**	**1.3/1.3**	**400/400**	**95/75**
Lunchmeat, salami (3 slices)	0	0.10	0.08	0.34	0
Macaroni and cheese (8 ounces)	48	0.25	0	0	0
Meat loaf (1 slice)	20	0.10	0.14	12	0.62
Melon, honeydew (1 cup)	5	0.07	0.16	34	32
Milk, fat-free (1 cup)	5	0.10	0.10	12	2
Milk, soy (1 cup)	0	0.15	0.16	40	0
Muffin, blueberry (1)	13	0.10	0.01	42	0.63
Mushrooms (1 cup sliced)	0	0.09	0.10	12	2
Nachos with cheese (6–8)	170	0.20	0.20	12	1
Nectarine (1)	23	0.05	0.03	7	7
Oatmeal (1 cup)	0.12	0.12	0.10	13	0
Olives (1 tablespoon)	1.70	0	0	0	0
Onion rings (10 medium)	0.98	0.10	0.07	64	0.68
Oyster (1 medium)	4.20	0.01	0.01	1.40	0.51
Pancakes (2)	7.60	0.16	0.07	28	0.15
Pasta with red sauce (4.5 ounces)	0	0.13	0.10	4	6
Peach (1 medium)	15	0.02	0.02	4	6
Peanut butter (2 tablespoons)	0	0.03	0.15	24	0
Peanuts (1 ounce)	0	0.12	0.07	41	0
Pear (1 medium)	1.60	0.02	0.05	12	7
Pepper, chile, raw (½ pepper)	21.6	0.03	0.23	10.35	65
Peppers, sweet (10 strips)	78	0.04	0.13	13	70
Pie, apple (1 piece)	37	0.03	0.04	32	4
Pizza, cheese (1 slice)	74	0.20	0.04	35	1
Pizza, vegetable (1 slice)	58	0.40	0.50	116	79
Plum (1)	21	0.03	0.05	1.45	6
Popcorn (1 cup)	0.80	0.02	0.02	2	0
Pork (3 ounces)	0	0.80	0.30	3	0
Potatoes, mashed (1 cup)	8.40	0.20	0.50	17	13
Potato salad (1 cup)	2.93	0.20	0.40	19	19
Potpie, chicken	256	0.30	0.20	41	2

VITAMIN E (MG)	CALCIUM (MG)	MAGNESIUM (MG)	POTASSIUM (MG)	SELENIUM (MCG)	ZINC (MG)	CALORIES
15/15	**1,000/1,000**	**420/320**	**4,700/4,700**	**55/55**	**11/8**	–
0.05	1.34	2.86	63	4	0.54	150
0	102	0	111	0	0	415
0.10	43	22	295	0	4	231
0.04	11	18	403	1.24	0.15	61
0.10	301	27	406	5	1	83
0	80	60	440	3	0.90	100
0.47	32	9	70	6	0.30	158
0.10	5	10	355	8	0.70	15
0	311	63	196	18	2	296
1	8	12	273	0	0.23	70
0.26	19	51	175	0	1.43	150
0.14	7	0.30	0.67	0.08	0	10
0.39	86	19	152	3	0.41	370
0.12	6	7	22	9	13	41
0.65	96	15	133	10	0.30	173
1.40	41	13	207	11	0.66	216
0.70	6	9	186	0.10	0.17	70
.0	12	51	214	2	1	190
.2	15	50	186	2	1	165
0.20	15	12	198	0.17	0.17	100
0.30	6	10	145	0.20	0.12	2
0.36	7	6.46	105	0	0	5
1.78	13	8	76	1	0.20	296
0	117	16	113	13	1	272
2	189	65	548	23	2	170
0	3	5	114	0.30	0.07	40
0	1	11	24	0.80	0.30	31
0.20	6	15	253	14	2	191
0.04	46	38	621	2	0.60	201
0.14	14	36	551	10	0.60	358
4	33	24	256	0.70	1	484

	VITAMIN A (MCG)	VITAMIN B1 (THIAMIN) (MG)	VITAMIN B6 (MG)	FOLATE (MCG)	VITAMIN C (MG)
RDA (men/women)	**900/700**	**1.2/1.1**	**1.3/1.3**	**400/400**	**95/75**
Pretzels (10 twists)	0	0.30	0.07	103	0
Raisins (1.5 ounces)	0	0.05	0.08	1.28	2.30
Raspberries (10)	0.38	0.01	0.01	4	5
Rice, brown (1 cup)	0	0.20	0.30	8	0
Rice, white (1 cup)	0	0.03	0.15	5	0
Ricotta cheese, part skim (½ cup)	132	0.03	0.02	16	0
Salad dressing, light Italian (1 tablespoon)	0	0	0	0	0
Salmon (3 ounces)	9.84	0.20	0.71	22	0
Salsa (½ cup)	44	0.05	0.16	21	18
Sauerkraut (1 cup)	1.42	0.03	0.18	34	21
Sausage (1 link)	0	0.05	0.01	0.26	0
Shrimp (4 large)	0	0.01	0.03	0.77	0.48
Soft drink with caffeine (12 ounces)	0	0	0	0	0
Soup, cream of chicken (1 cup)	179	0.07	0.07	7	1.24
Soup, tomato (1 cup)	29.28	0.09	0.11	15	66
Soybeans (1 cup cooked)	14	0.47	0.10	200	31
Spaghetti with meatballs (1½ cups)	46	0.38	0.43	101	24
Spareribs (3 ounces)	1.91	0.26	0.22	3	0
Spinach (1 cup)	140	0.02	0.06	58	8
Steak (different cuts)	0	0.10	0.30	6	0
Strawberries (1 cup)	1.66	0.03	0.09	40	97
Submarine sandwich	71	1	0.10	87	12
Sunflower seeds (1/4 cup)	6	0	0.28	82	0.50
Sweet potato (1)	350	0.09	0.25	9	19
Taco salad (1.5 cups)	71	0.10	0.20	83	4
Toaster pastry (1)	148	0.20	0.20	15	0
Tofu (4 ounces)	4.96	0.10	0.06	19	0
Tomato (1 medium)	26	0.02	0.05	9	8
Tuna salad (1 cup)	49	0.06	0.17	16	5
Turkey, skinless (½ breast)	0	0.16	2.26	31	0
Vegetable juice (1 cup)	188	0.10	0.30	51	67

VITAMIN E (MG)	CALCIUM (MG)	MAGNESIUM (MG)	POTASSIUM (MG)	SELENIUM (MCG)	ZINC (MG)	CALORIES
15/15	**1,000/1,000**	**420/320**	**4,700/4,700**	**55/55**	**11/8**	**–**
0.21	22	21	88	3	0.50	229
0.30	12	13	350	0.26	0.08	127
0.17	5	4	28	0.04	0.08	10
0.06	20	84	84	19	1	216
0.06	16	19	55	12	0.80	205
0.09	337	19	155	21	1.70	171
0	0	0	2	0.20	0	26
0.95	11	28	475	35	0.60	175
1.53	39	17	275	0.50	0.30	41
0.14	43	18	241	0.90	0.30	45
0.03	1.30	1.56	25	1.87	0.24	125
0	9	7	40	9	0.30	22
0	10	3	3	0.34	0	154
0.25	181	17	272	8	0.67	225
2	12	7	263	0.50	0.24	180
0.02	261	108	970	3	1.64	298
4	138	66	718	39	5	545
0.20	30	15	204	24	3	338
0.60	30	24	167	0.30	0.16	10
0.11	4	19	250	12	3.26	217
0.50	27	22	253	1	0.20	46
0	189	68	394	31	2.60	386
12	42	127	248	21.42	1.82	205
1.42	41	27	348	0.30	0.30	103
192	51	416	4	3	0	279
0.90	17	12	57	6.30	0.30	204
0.01	434	37	150	11	1	75
0.33	6	7	146	0	0.11	35
2	35	39	365	84	1	383
0.30	39	109	1,142	95	5	413
12	26	27	467	1	0.50	50

	VITAMIN A (MCG)	VITAMIN B1 (THIAMIN) (MG)	VITAMIN B6 (MG)	FOLATE (MCG)	VITAMIN C (MG)
RDA (men/women)	**900/700**	**1.2/1.1**	**1.3/1.3**	**400/400**	**95/75**
Walnuts (1 cup)	37	0.27	0.70	82	4
Watermelon (1 wedge)	104	0.20	0.40	6	31
Wheat germ (½ cup)	0	0.20	0.40	81	0
Whey protein powder (2 teaspoons)	0	0	0	0	0
Wine, red (3.5 ounces)	0	0	0.03	2	0
Wine, white (3.5 ounces)	0	0	0.01	0	0
Yogurt, low-fat (8 ounces)	2	0.10	0.09	24	1.70

VITAMIN E (MG)	CALCIUM (MG)	MAGNESIUM (MG)	POTASSIUM (MG)	SELENIUM (MCG)	ZINC (MG)	CALORIES
15/15	**1,000/1,000**	**420/320**	**4,700/4,700**	**55/55**	**11/8**	**–**
0	73	253	655	21	4.28	654
0.40	41	31	479	0.30	0.20	86
0	27	275	166	91	14	104
0	0	0	260	0	0	21
0	8	13	111	0.20	0.10	88
0	9	10	80	0.20	0.07	86
0	415	37	497	11	1.88	193

APPENDIX D

Glycemic Loads for Selected Foods

HOW TO USE THIS CHART: The numbers in this chart represent the glycemic loads (GLs) of common foods. The GL is the product of a food's glycemic index and the amount of carbohydrates available per serving. Essentially, the GL estimates the projected elevation in blood glucose caused by eating a particular food. The higher a food's GL, the more likely it is to raise your blood sugar, and the higher it will likely be in calories and carbs. Try to focus on foods with a GL of 19 or less, and shoot for a total GL of less than 120 per day if you decide to count.

Food	GL
Peanuts	1
Low-fat yogurt, artificially sweetened	2
Carrots	3
Grapefruit	3
Green peas	3
Fat-free milk	4
Pear	4
Watermelon	4
Beets	5
Orange	5
Peach	5
Plum	5
Apple	6
Kiwifruit	6
Tomato soup	6
Baked beans	7
Chickpeas, canned	7
Grapes	7
Pineapple	7
Whole wheat bread	7
Popcorn	8
Soy milk	8
Taco shells	8
All-Bran cereal	9
Grapefruit juice	9
Hamburger bun	9
Kidney beans, canned	9
Lentil soup	9
Oatmeal cookies	9
Sweet corn	9
American rye bread	10
Cheese tortellini	10
Frozen waffles	10

Honey	10	Blueberry muffin	17
Lima beans, frozen	10	Corn chips	17
Low-fat yogurt, sweetened with sugar	10	Doughnut	17
		Grape-Nuts Flakes cereal	17
Pinto beans	10	Instant oatmeal	17
White bread	10	Rice cakes	17
Bran Chex cereal	11	Sweet potato	17
Apple juice	12	Total cereal	17
Banana	12	Brown rice	18
Kaiser roll	12	Fettuccine	18
Orange juice	12	Angel food cake	19
Saltine crackers	12	Cornflakes cereal	21
Bran flakes	13	French fries	22
Oatmeal	13	Jelly beans	22
Graham crackers	14	Macaroni	22
Special K cereal	14	Rice Krispies cereal	22
Vanilla wafers	14	Couscous	23
Bran muffin	15	Linguine	23
Cheerios cereal	15	Long-grain rice	23
French bread	15	White rice	23
Grape-Nuts cereal	15	Bagel	25
Mashed potatoes	15	Baked potato	26
Shredded wheat cereal	15	Spaghetti	27
Bread stuffing mix	16	Raisins	28
Cheese pizza	16	Macaroni and cheese	32
Whole wheat spaghetti	16	Instant rice	36
Black bean soup	17		

APPENDIX E
Conversion Charts

VOLUME MEASUREMENTS

U.S.	IMPERIAL	METRIC
¼ teaspoon	n/a	1 ml
½ teaspoon	n/a	2 ml
1 teaspoon	n/a	5 ml
1 tablespoon	n/a	15 ml
2 tablespoons (1 oz)	1 fl oz	30 ml
¼ cup (2 oz)	2 fl oz	60 ml
⅓ cup (3 oz)	3 fl oz	80 ml
½ cup (4 oz)	4 fl oz	120 ml
⅔ cup (5 oz)	5 fl oz	160 ml
¾ cup (6 oz)	6 fl oz	180 ml
1 cup (8 oz)	8 fl oz	240 ml

WEIGHT MEASUREMENTS

U.S.	METRIC
1 oz	30 g
2 oz	60 g
4 oz	115 g
5 oz	145 g
6 oz	170 g
7 oz	200 g
8 oz	230 g
10 oz	285 g
12 oz	340 g
14 oz	400 g
16 oz	455 g
2.2 1b	1 kg

LENGTH MEASUREMENTS

U.S.	METRIC
¼"	0.6 cm
½"	1.25 cm
1"	2.5 cm
2"	5 cm
4"	11 cm
6"	15 cm
8"	20 cm
10"	25 cm
12"	30 cm

These equivalents have been slightly rounded to make measuring easier.

PAN SIZES

U.S.	METRIC
8" cake pan	20 x 4 cm sandwich or cake tin
9" cake pan	23 x 3.5 cm sandwich or cake tin
11" x 17" baking pan	28 x 18 cm baking tin
13" x 9" baking pan	32.5 x 23 cm baking tin
15" x 10" baking pan	38 x 23 cm baking tin (Swiss roll tin)
1½ qt baking dish	1.5 liter baking dish
2 qt rectangular baking dish	30 x 19 cm baking dish
9" pie plate	22 x 4 or 23 x 4 cm pie plate
7" or 8" springform pan	18 or 20 cm springform or loose-bottom cake tin
9" x 5" loaf pan	23 x 13 cm or 2 lb narrow loaf tin or pâté tin

TEMPERATURES

FAHRENHEIT	CELSIUS
140°	60°
160°	70°
180°	80°
225°	105°
250°	120°
275°	135°
300°	150°
325°	160°
350°	180°
375°	190°
400°	200°
425°	220°
450°	230°
475°	245°
500°	260°

INDEX

<u>Underscored</u> page references indicate boxed text. **Boldfaced** page references indicate photographs.